The HALO Affect

The HALO Affect

Tim Atkinson's **H**igh **A**ctivity **L**ow **O**besity
Diet and Exercise Plan

A Practical Approach to Weight Reduction and Weight Management Based on Scientific Understanding of Fat and Body Weight Regulation

Tim Atkinson

iUniverse, Inc.
New York Lincoln Shanghai

The HALO Affect
Tim Atkinson's High Activity Low Obesity Diet and Exercise Plan

iUniverse books may be ordered through booksellers or by contacting:

iUniverse
2021 Pine Lake Road, Suite 100
Lincoln, NE 68512
www.iuniverse.com
1-800-Authors (1-800-288-4677)

ISBN: 0-595-34916-1

Printed in the United States of America

CONTENTS

PREFACE

The purpose of this book is to provide a scientific basis to the understanding of dieting and weight gain and to explain why we get fat based on nutritional, psychological, and sports science evidence. It has combined scientific data with anecdotal and personal experience to illustrate overweight and obesity susceptibility and why we need to proactively address weight management to stave off disease and ill health.

The book has been created as an educational tool to help people to help themselves. It is certainly true that knowledge is power and, with the right ingredients, people can stop the habitualisation of overeating and manage their food intake in a healthy balanced way.

I hope that the book will inspire and educate those who not only have weight issues but those who simply want to become healthier through a reasoned approach to health and weight management.

CHAPTER 1

The Origins of Fat

We are all getting fatter! This is perhaps the only undisputed consensus that has emerged from the medical and media communities over recent years. Unfortunately, this worrying trend is set to continue well into the 21st Century—The International Obesity Task Force has stated that obesity has increased 10-40% in the majority of European countries in the past 10 years, and the American Obesity Assocation states that approximately 127 million adults in the US are overweight, made up of 60 million obese people and 9 million severely obese. Today, about 64% of all adult Americans are obese, a figure that is expected to increase with simultaneous increases throughout Europe and and the rest of the world.

So what is our problem with weight gain? Why are we all becoming overweight and obese? Is it pathological? Or is it habitual? Do our genes play a role? Is it caused by a virus? Are we predestined to become fat or is gluttony prevailing? Although these questions remain to be answered by academic research scientists who may ponder on biochemistry and human genetics, there are simpler explanations to our rapidly expanding waistlines. Some may say, for obvious reasons, that the readily available and universally marketed supply of fast food, which is high in fats, sugars and salt, is to blame, in addition to increased snacking due to lack of time and habitual behaviours, and the fact that people do not do enough exercise because of preferred sedentary lifestyles. All are valid points to make, which tends to suggest our time-urgent lifestyles demand prompt access to, and delivery of, hassle-free quick-fix food, without the chore of cooking and clearing up—analogous to disposable goods where all the work is done in terms of manufacturing and packaging. Put succinctly, all we need to do is open our mouths, throw in the food, chew, swallow, then throw away the packaging. However, this disposable ready-made culture has become a way of life for many of us trying to balance the work-home scales and has rapidly become the norm in many nations.

It is unsurprising then that media attention has, in recent years, focused on food and our relationship with body weight through countless magazines, television shows, books, work-out DVDs and CDs. In addition, the obesity pandemic has sparked a frenzy of healty eating campaigns, health fads, diets, and supplements which are cleverly marketed to target our consumer obsession with calories, carbohydrates, fats, and sugar levels. Although overeating and a lack of exercise may account for part of the probem in overweight, there has to be another reason why some of us become fatter yet others do not.

Why do some people get fat and others do not?

If a sample of 100 randomly picked people were given 6 healthy meals a day for 6 weeks (3 times more than the average meals per day) there would be a good chance that some would put on weight whereas others would merely maintain their weight even if the calorific intake was the same for all participants during every meal. This is because we are all genetically different and our biology dictates what we eat and how we eat it. For example, those who were used to eating more than three meals a day, through snacking for example, would probably have no problem accommodating more food and may be prone to gaining weight; those with a smaller appetite however may restrict food intake and not eat all the food freely available so they may keep a constant weight. Furthermore, there may be a genetic propensity for individuals to eat more sugary or fatty foods than others so these individuals would be at liberty to increase their intake of these foods and tend to gain weight. In contrast, those who favour savoury foods and avoid foods high in fat and sugar may regulate their body weight more effectively in the presence of excessive food availability. These are just a few of the many examples why some people become fatter whilst others do not. Our biological make up plays an enormous part in how we function, how we eat, how much we eat, how food is stored, how it is expended and how it is excreted.

The key to understanding our weight gain is held in the understanding of the mechanisms of food intake and regulation, which occurs in the brain. Although it is far from clear how weight regulation actually works medical and scientific evidence suggests that being overweight and obesity results from a variety of causes including dysfunctional biological mediators of weight regulation, a genetic predisposition to fatness, natural ageing, sociocultural and/or environmental influences, and the more commonly accepted notion of excessive dietary fat intake and low levels of physical activity, commensurate with affluent industrialised lifestyles.

So what is fat?

Fats are made up of fatty acids which are chemical compounds that exist as either saturated, polyunsaturated or monounsaturated fats. Dietary fats may be saturated (animal) or unsaturated (vegetable) in origin and include butter, margarine, cream, milk, nuts, and red meats. Low fat dietary intake is known to lower blood cholesterol levels—cholesterol is a type of fat that causes heart disease in high concentrations—whereas high total fat intake will increase cholesterol levels and potentially cause an increase in body weight and the risk of heart disease. Interestingly, 'obesity' is derived from the Latin word 'obesus' which means fat or plump. Similarly, the Greek expression 'ob-edere' means intensive (ob) eating (edere).

In understanding weight gain, we need to look at food intake, both volume and quality of food, and the relationship between appetite and energy expenditure. To start this let us take a look at obesity. Medical scientists have conducted years of research into obesity, a condition characterised by excessive body fat. It results from an imbalance between energy intake and energy expenditure. So, this cause-effect relationship means that if we do not burn off the energy through physical activity, fat will be stored by the body thereby increasing body weight. The exact cause(s) of obesity are unclear but genetic, physiological, metabolic, nutritional, environmental, and behavioural factors may all contribute to its progression into a long-term and lifelong condition. Furthermore, it is associated with serious comorbidities such as coronary heart disease, hypertension, non-insulin-dependent diabetes mellitus (NIDDM), and dyslipidaemia making it a public health epidemic.

Being overweight is not necessarily an indication of obesity, but if your body mass index (BMI) (a simple index of weight-for-height and is commonly used worldwide for denoting the classification of obesity in adults) is over 30, it is now widely accepted as denoting obesity.

A BMI is calculated as the weight in kilograms divided by the square of the height in metres (kg/m^2): BMI = weight (kg)/$height^2$(m)

However if you are overweight and your cholesterol levels are high it means that there is an increased risk of heart disease and a susceptibility to increased weight further. Generally, men who have more than 25% body fat and women with more than 35% body fat are considered obese. Fat distribution in these individuals usually takes two forms: central abdominal or android obesity (apples) and gluteofemoral or gynoid obesity (pears). Android obesity (typical of men) can be distinguished from gynoid obesity (typical of women) by calculating a waist-to-hip ratio (WHR). A WHR of 0.8 or lower is usually found in women and a WHR of 0.85 or higher is usually found in men. A waist circumference that exceeds 102 cm (40 inches) in men or 97 cm (38 inches) in women is sometimes considered to be android obesity, but this has little significance as it does not take into account an individual's height or large bone structure.

Additionally, the distribution as well as amount of fat has other health implications: central abdominal fat is shown to be the major contributor to insulin resistance and risk of diabetes, hypertension and cardiovascular disease.

Am I obese?

The international BMI classification of overweight and obesity according to the World Health Organisation is shown in Table 1.1. This classification includes an additional subdivision at BMI 35.0-39.9 in recognition that management options for dealing with obesity differ above a BMI of 35 (Table 1.2).

Table 1.0 Standard table of Body Mass Index

	5'0"	5'3"	5'6"	5'9"	6'0"	6'3"
140	27	25	23	21	19	18
150	29	27	24	22	20	19
160	31	28	26	24	22	20
170	33	30	28	25	23	21
180	35	32	29	27	25	23
190	37	34	31	28	26	24
200	39	36	32	30	27	25
210	41	37	34	31	29	26
220	43	39	36	33	30	28
230	45	41	37	34	31	29
240	47	43	39	36	33	30
250	49	44	40	37	34	31

Table 1.2: WHO classification of overweight in adults according to BMI

Classification	BMI (kg/m^2)	Risk of comorbidities
Underweight	<18.5	Low (but risk of other clinical problems increased)
Normal range	18.5-24.9	Average
Overweight	≥25	
Pre-obese	25.0-29.9	Increased
Obese class I	30.0-34.9	Moderate
Obese class II	35.0-39.9	Severe
Obese class III	≥40.0	Very severe

Source: WHO, 1997

CHAPTER 2

What Causes Fatness?

Being overweight and obese is a complex condition involving many physiological, psychological and environmental factors. According to some experts there is unlikely to be a one single theory to explain its occurrence. On the premise that obesity has been studied extensively over the past 30 years, we can use research data from its study to make some associations and putative links to why we increase our weight.

Evidence that obesity is a complex disorder with a variety of causes comes from scientific research studies in the following areas:

- Neurology
- Endocrinology
- Molecular genetics
- Metabolism
- Biochemistry
- Physiology
- Nutrition
- Physical activity
- Psychosocial/behavioural psychology
- Environment

To grasp an understanding of how mechanisms in these different disciplines work together to increase body weight we must look at normal body weight regulation first.

What is normal body weight regulation?

Normal body weight regulation (how our bodies keep a balance of what goes in and what comes out) is determined and controlled by the relationships between (1) external and environmental factors (such as eating behaviour, composition of foods, and physical activity); (2) internal physiological processes (such as neuroendocrine control of appetite, metabolic and bio-chemical aspects of energy intake and expenditure, and (3) molecular genetics (including the molecular mechanisms of adipose or fat tissue production and regulation within the body).

Obesity and being overweight develops when any one or more of the processes associated with these interactions, or the interactions themselves, are either increased or decreased or stopped altogether, resulting in increased energy intake (more food going in) and decreased energy expenditure (more food being stored as fat and sugar).

What are the forces at work to destabilise the normal regulation of food intake?

Age and Gender

The first force at work is natural ageing. This plays a part in the processes lead-ing to overweight. As a general rule, the older you are, the slower the metabolic rate of the body. Therefore, if one compared the weight of a person at 40 years of age to when they were 20 years of age taking into account that the diet and physical activities were constant for both, there is a greater chance that the per-son at 40 years of age will have gained weight.

Also, the rate of formation and storage of new fat cells or adipocytes is faster in the first few years of life. In obese children, for example, the number of fat cells is often as much as three times that in normal children. After adolescence, the number of adipocytes remain almost identical throughout life; therefore it has been suggested that overfeeding of children can predispose them to a lifetime of being overweight and obesity.

Gender is also an important factor. Men have a higher resting metabolic rate (RMR) than women and so require more calories to maintain their body weight. Additionally, when women become postmenopausal, their metabolic rate decreases significantly, which is why they are prone to weight gain post menopause.

The Biology

Hunger and satiety

Eating is a complex behaviour involving numerous physiological and psychological factors and interactions. Normal food intake is controlled by the lateral hypothalamus of the brain, which is also known as the appetite centre. This area motivates the individual to actively search for food and eat. In the ventromedial portion of the hypothalamus, a satiety centre (the part that makes us feel full) acts to inhibit appetite when adequate food intake has been achieved. Higher centres than the hypothalamus also play important roles in the control of feeding, particularly the amygdala and some cortical areas of the limbic system. These brain areas are involved in the modulation of eating patterns. The mechanism of food regulation and energy balance involves a complex signalling network between neuroanatomical structures, hormones, neurotransmitters, and peptide receptors. It includes the coordination of signals to the brain of taste perception and memory at times of feeding, signals of fat mass at a tissue level, and signals from the gastrointestinal tract related to the presence of food and the digestive process.

At this cellular level, abnormal body weight regulation occurs when the central mechanisms that control food intake and energy balance are disturbed or damaged. However, at a conscious level, these control mechanisms might be influenced by sociocultural, psychological and environmental aspects of eating and lifestyle activities. Although we cannot alter the internal mechanics of weight regulation we can act on those mechanisms that are sociocultural, psychological, and environmental—the basis for the HALO Diet and Activity Plan.

Neurological and endocrinological abnormalities and weight gain

Evidence to suggest that weight gain and obesity can be caused by physiological abnormalities comes from a number of endocrinological and neurological conditions. The most common are listed in Table 1.3.

Table 1.3 Neurological and endocrinological disorders associated with ovweweight and obesity

Disorder	Relation to overweight and obesity
Hypothyroidism	Weight gain results as a consequence of decreased energy expenditure
Disorders of corticosteroid metabolism, e.g Cushing's syndrome	Weight gain accompanied by characteristic patterns of fat deposition in the truncal region
Sex hormone disorders, e.g Hypogonadism; ovariectomy	Causes increases in energy intake and weight gain
Other hormone disorders, e.g Insulinoma; growth hormone deficiency	Causes increases in energy intake and weight gain
Polycystic ovarian syndrome	Altered ovarian function or hypersensitivity of the hypothalamic-pituitary-adrenal axis resulting in hormonally induced weight gain
Hypothalamic tumour Brain damage to hypothalamic region Brain infection Brain trauma	Results in a defect in appetite control and subsequent hyperphagia
Congenital abnormalities e.g Prader-Willi syndrome	Hypothalamic defect resulting in hyperphagia

Source: Adapted from Jebb, 1997

Are genetics involved?

In animal models, single defect genes have been identified that can lead to obesity. Human obesity, however, is more complex than comparative animal models of obesity and because it is a disorder with no single cause, single gene defects are more difficult to identify. Nevertheless, small populations of genetically determined conditions have resulted in excess weight and fatness (eg Prader-Willi syndrome; Bardet-Biedl syndrome; Cohen's syndrome; Simpson-Golabi-Behmel syndrome; Carpenter's syndrome) but these account for only a small proportion of the obese population. Geneticists have recently provided an update on the human obesity gene map documenting an increase from three single obesity gene mutations in two genes in 1997, to 25 cases due to 12 mutations in seven genes in 1999.

Animal studies

During the past decade scientists have cloned a number of genes associated with single-gene defects causing overweight and obesity in mice (Table 1.4).

Table 1.4: Genetic models of obesity in mice

Single-gene mutations	Gene product
Ob/ob	OB protein (leptin)
Db/db	OB receptor
Fat/fat	Carboxypeptidase E
Tub/tub	TUB protein
Agouti	AGOUTI protein
Mg/mg	Mahogany protein
PTP-1B	Protein tyrosine phosphatase -1B
β_3 *adrenoceptor*	β_3 adrenoceptor

Source: Adapted from Grippo and Burn, 1998.

Let us look in more detail at scientific animal studies to see if genetics play a role in being overweight and obese.

agouti

The earliest mouse obesity gene, called *agouti,* was cloned by Bultman *et al.,* in 1992. Too much agouti protein produced a condition in mice characterised by a yellow coat, obesity, hyperinsulinaemia and hyperglycaemia (Klebig *et al.,* 1995)

ob/ob

First characterised in 1950 as the first recessive obesity mutation discovered, the *ob* gene—cloned in 1994—caused ob/ob mice to exhibit severe early onset obesity, insulin resistance and strain susceptibility to diabetes, a combination resembling morbid obesity in humans (Zhang *et al.,* 1994). This discovery had a remarkable impact on research into obesity because it was found that a deficiency in the gene product (OB protein or leptin), which is synthesised and secreted by adipocytes, was suggested to be the cause of the obese condition in the *ob/ob* mice. Investigators confirmed this by demonstrating that injections of leptin into *ob/ob* mice reduced food consumption, body weight, per cent fat, serum glucose and insulin (Pellymounter *et al.,* 1995). Additional studies (Campfield *et al.,* 1995; Halaas *et al.,* 1995) confirmed this weight regulation effect in ob/ob animals suggesting that a circulating protein-based signal generated from adipocytes can act on central neuronal networks. It was also shown that in diet-induced obese mice, leptin reduced food intake and body weight indicating a possible therapeutic role for leptin in human obesity (Campfield *et al.,* 1995). The leptin receptor has also been cloned (Tartaglia *et al.,* 1995).

db/db

The *db* mouse gene and its human homologue were first cloned in 1995 by Tartaglia (Tartaglia *et al.,* 1995). Mice with the *db* gene express almost the same phenotype as *ob/ob* mice. However, injections of leptin did not reduce food intake and weight loss suggesting that a defect is present in the receptor that mediates the action of leptin. It was subsequently found that these mice display leptin receptor mutations that result in defects in molecular signalling (Chen *et al.*, 1996; Lee *et al.*, 1996; Chua *et al.*, 1996).

fat/fat

Obesity develops at a slower pace in *fat/fat* mice compared with *ob/ob* or *db/db* mice but can be up to two to three times heavier than wild-type litter mates (Keightley, 1995). The gene product, carboxypeptidase E protein (CPE), was found to be mutated in *fat/fat* mice (Naggert *et al.*, 1995). CPE is involved in the processing of a number of prohormones and possibly influences the biochemical pathway of hormones and receptors in the brain involved with food intake and weight control.

tub/tub

Mice with the *tub* gene develop obesity despite consuming a normal amount of food; they go on to develop hyperinsulinaemia and impaired glucose tolerance. The *tub* gene product was discovered in 1995 (Noben-Trauth K, *et al.*, 1996; Kleyn PW *et al.*, 1996) but to-date the tub protein remains a mystery in the metabolic pathway of obesity.

ob, db, fat, and agouti

Studies have suggested that all four known mutations lie within the same biochemical pathway linking leptin secreted from adipocytes to the activation of weight-regulating melanocortin-4 (MC-4) receptors in the brain (Seeley *et al.*, 1997; Schwartz *et al.*, 1997; Thiele *et al.*, 1998)

β_3-adrenoceptor

A mutation in the β_3-adrenoceptor gene was found to be phenotypically responsible for a low resting metabolic rate in humans and is now linked to obesity (Walston *et al* 1995; Liu *et al.*, 1995).

mg

The *mahogany* (*mg*) gene (Nagle *et al.*,1999) product, MG protein, was found to be mainly active in the area of the hypothalamus, which is associated with body weight regulation. Mice with a normal *mg* gene gain excess weight on a high fat diet, whereas mutant *mg/mg* mice maintained a healthy weight when fed a high fat or low fat diet. Although researchers are unsure about how the MG protein works, it is believed that the molecule either functions as a transport protein that blocks the function of certain weight-regulating melanocortin receptors, thus enhancing the receptors' signalling, or that the protein may be a signalling receptor involved in food and weight regulation.

Protein tyrosine phosphatase-1B gene

The protein tyrosine phosphatase-1B (PTP-1B) gene, the gene product of which is an enzyme involved in the regulation of insulin—has been linked to obesity and insulin insensitivity (Kennedy *et al*, 1999). Researchers have shown that PTP-1B 'knockout' mice—those with the gene genetically knocked out cancelling its production—were resistant to weight gain and remained insulin sensitive, whereas normal mice rapidly gained weight and became insulin resistant when both groups were fed a high-fat diet. The investigators suggest that because fat metabolism has been affected in the knockout animals, PTP-1B might become the basis of a new treatment for obesity and NIDDM.

How does this relate to human weight gain and obesity

Because not enough research has been conducted on humans we cannot make any generalisations to human weight gain, but the animal research does tell us that there may indeed be a genetic association to weight gain. Although researchers believe that our genes are associated with adipose tissue production and may cause overweight and obesity, the true genetic basis for human obesity is not yet known.

These genes of interest include hormone sensitive lipase, beta-2 and beta-3-adrenoceptors, tumour necrosis factor-alpha, low-density lipoprotein receptor, uncoupling protein-1 and peroxisome-proliferator activated receptor gamma-2. These genes may also promote obesity by gene-gene interactions (eg. beta-3-adrenoceptors and uncoupling protein-1) or gene-environmental interactions (eg. beta-2-adrenoceptors and physical activity).

Maybe its my metabolism that causes me to become overweight?

Many people do use the argument that they are overweight because they believe it has something to do with their metabolic rate. Indeed, metabolic predictors of body weight gain have been identified from cross-sectional studies of obese and lean individuals. Generally, metabolic factors of weight gain include:

- Low resting metabolic rate (LRMR)
- Low level of physical activity
- Substrate oxidation rates
- Thermogenic activity levels

Let us look in detail at these factors.

Resting metabolic rate

Since 1992, the National Institutes of Health (NIH) in the USA has studied a population of Pima Indians in Phoenix, Arizona, USA, to investigate risk factors associated with the development of NIDDM and obesity. It was found that Indians with low RMR were approximately eight times more at risk of gaining 10 kg of body weight compared with those with a high RMR (Ravussin *et al.*, 1988; Roberts *et al.*, 1988; Griffiths *et al.*, 1990).

RMR generally represents 60% of daily energy expenditure and depends largely on fat-free body mass, which is more metabolically active than fat tissue (Nelson *et al.*, 1992). Therefore, overweight and obese people generally have higher RMR than lean people because of the increased body size including fat-free mass. However, researchers have found fat-free mass and RMR to be comparable for both obese and nonobese individuals after adjustment for body composition (Bogardus *et al.*, 1986; Nelson *et al.*, 1992; Ravussin *et al.*, 1988) suggesting that there is variability in RMR among individuals.

It is assumed, therefore, that a low RMR was associated with weight gain and several longitudinal studies addressed this possibility: one study (Seidell *et al.*, 1992) found no association of baseline RMR with weight change; another (Weinsier *et al.*, 1995) found that RMR did not predict weight gain although obesity prone women gained significantly more weight over a 4-year follow-up period; furthermore, a low RMR was not a significant predictor of weight gain during a 2-4 year follow-up period (Ravussin *et al.*, 1988); and other data (Goran *et al.*, 1998) indicated that initial RMR did not predict changes in fat mass in children followed up for 4 years. It can be deduced therefore that normal variations in body-composition-adjusted RMR may affect daily energy requirements, but that they will only have a small impact on one's tendency to gain weight (Weinsier *et al.*, 1988).

Contrary to these studies, a relatively low total daily energy expenditure has been found to be strongly correlated with weight gain (Ravussin *et al.*, 1988) and this was confirmed in other investigations where spontaneous activity related energy expenditure was observed (Zurlo *et al.*, 1992; Goran 1995; Carpenter *et al.*, 1995). In simple terms this could mean that, as a component of total daily energy expenditure, a reduced activity-related metabolic rate might predispose an individual to being overweight and obese.

Physical activity and metabolism

There is strong association between physical activity and weight gain. In a large population survey of over 12000 Finnish adults, overweight was found to be much higher in sedentary (inactive) women (21%) and men (14%) compared with physically active women (8%) and men (7%) (Rissanen *et al.*, 1991). Obesity experts in the UK have suggested that a modern inactive lifestyle plays an important role in the increasing prevalence of obesity (Prentice & Jebb, 1995). Support for the role of physical inactivity in the development of obesity comes from a study where normal weight postobese women who reported being 'nonexercisers' gained more than twice as much weight over 4 years of follow-up than those who excercised regularly (Weinsier *et al.*, 1995).

Thermogenesis

Thermogenesis is the production of heat during the chemical process of fat oxidation. Fat oxidation is when fat is burned up to be used as energy during body tissue respiration and accounts for only a fraction of total energy expenditure but a defect in the process is thought by some to account for the development of overweight and obesity. A number of studies suggest that an increase in energy expenditure after food is possibly due to a decreased sympathetic nervous sytstem (SNS) activity (Astrup *et al.*, 1987). The SNS is a major physiological regulator of body homeostasis. It regulates the cardiovascular system and blood pressure but also has an important role in regulating body temperature, digestive secretions, respiratory function and pupillary dilation. Additionally, the SNS has effects on the pancreas and adipose tissue. Animal studies have shown that low SNS activity predisposes to obesity via thermogenesis (Niijima *et al.*, 1984) but large inconsistencies are found in the literature when SNS activity is compared in lean and obese humans (Tataranni 1998). However, a logitudinal analysis in Pima Indians shows that low SNS activity is associated with body weight gain and central adiposity (Tataranni *et al.*, 1997).

Does our biochemistry cause a propensity to being overweight and obese?

Many biochemicals are involved in the regulation of body weight. These include: neurotransmitters in the brain that act on the appetite centre; hormones that affect food intake and regulation; signal transporter proteins and receptors involved in the metabolic pathway of weight regulation; and enzymes involved in the metabolism of nutrients. Experts suggest that there are probably hundreds or even thousands of other gene products and molecules that have not yet been discovered, which contribute to the pathophysiology of obesity (Bessesen & Faggioni, 1998). Arguably, defects in any one or more of the peptides might interfere with the normal intake of food and body weight regulation and these peptide molecules have to-date been the focus of pharmacological antiobesity treatments. Protein molecules commonly associated with food intake and regulation are listed in Table 1.5.

Table 1.5 Protein associated with food intake and body weight regulation

Function	Protein molecule	
	Increase food intake	Decrease food intake
Neurotransmitters	Noradrenaline Opioid Growth hormone releasing hormone Galanin Neuropeptide Y Melanin-concentrating hormone	Serotonin Dopamine Cholecystokinin Corticotrophin-releasing factor Neurotensin Bombesin Amylin Adrenomedullin Glucagon Glucagon-like peptide-1
Pancreatic hormone		Insulin
Glucocorticoids		Cortisol Cortisone
Fat-derived hormone		Leptin
Enzyme	PTP-1B	

Animal studies indicate that the most potent neuropeptides that might play a critical role in influencing energy balance include neuropeptide Y (NPY), corticotrophin-releasing hormone (CRH), glucagon-like peptide 1 (GLP-1), insulin, and leptin. Many other neuropeptides and hormone signalling molecules and receptors are, however, also implicated in the normal regulation of food intake and maintenance of body weight, but a selection of peptides commonly associated with overweight and obesity is discussed below:

Neuropeptide Y

NPY is found in high concentrations in the hypothalamus of the brain and induces feeding by interacting with a receptor subtype that binds NPY (O'Shea et al., 1997). Injections of NPY into the paraventricular nucleus of the brain reduces energy expenditure by inhibiting the sympathetic nerves that innervate and stimulate brown adipose tissue (BAT), causing hyperphagia (Billington et al., 1991). NPY is the only neurotransmitter that when given as a repeated dose will increase body fat and induce true obesity, an effect also observed in satiated animals (Paez et al., 1991).

Carboxypeptidase E

Carboxypeptidase E (CPE) is an enzyme that may be involved in the final stages of processing insulin, pro-opiomelanocortin (POMC), and other hormones. Interestingly, an obese person has been identified who carries a mutation in the gene for prohormone convertase-1 (PC-1), an enzyme that catalyzes a reaction preceding that catalyzed by CPE (Jackson 1997). These findings indicate that correct processing of certain, as yet unknown, proteins and hormones can be essential for mice and humans to maintain a lean body composition.

Corticotrophin-releasing hormone

CRH has the opposite effect to NPY. It stops feeding and increases metabolic rate when injected into the brains of animals. CRH reduces obesity through stimulation of sympathetic nerve-mediated mechanisms and inhibition of vagus nerve-mediated mechanisms (Thorburn & Proietto 1998). It also involved in the regulation of insulin, adrenocorticothrophic hormone and glucocorticoid production (Plotsky et al., 1992; Rohner-Jeanrenaud & Jeanrenaud 1992).

Glucagon-like peptide-1

GLP-1 is produced in the small intestine in response to mixed meals. It stimulates insulin secretion and inhibits gastrointestinal secretion and motility. Its dual function appears to signal nutritional abundance and enhances deposition of nutrients (Holst 1994). Its role in overweight and obesity was demonstrated when brain injections of GLP-1 inhibited feeding in rats (Turton *et al.*, 1996).

Insulin

Insulin, which is produced by the pancreas, is a hormone that promotes the conversion of glucose to fat and storage of fat in adipose tissue. Many obese subjects tend to be hyperinsulinaemic (high insulin levels)—perhaps because eating increases insulin secretion. Insulin injected centrally has the opposite effect on fat deposition to peripheral insulin injections. When administered into the hypothalamus of the brain, it inhibits feeding, stimulates BAT thermogenesis and causes weight loss (Schwartz *et al.*, 1992). Insulin is believed to affect food intake by reducing NPY expression in the hypothalamus (Sipols *et al.*, 1994).

Protein tyrosine phosphatase-1B

Protein tyrosine phosphatase-1B (PTP-1B), an enzyme involved in the regulation of insulin—has recently been linked to obesity and insulin insensitivity (Kennedy *et al*, 1999). Researchers have shown that mutated PTP-1B gene mice were resistant to weight gain and remained insulin sensitive, whereas normal mice rapidly gained weight and became insulin resistant when both groups were fed a high-fat diet. The investigators suggest that because fat metabolism has been affected in the knockout animals, PTP-1B might become the basis of a new treatment for obesity.

Leptin

Leptin is the gene product of the *ob* gene and is secreted by adipocytes or fat cells. Since its discovery in 1994, leptin deficiency and leptin resistance has been found to lead to severe obesity in mice, suggesting that it might be crucial to the normal control of food intake and body weight (Frühbeck *et al.* 1998). However, only a few cases of congenital leptin deficiency associated with severe early-onset obesity have been documented (Montague *et al.*, 1997; Strobel *et al.*, 1998). Strangely, most overweight and obese patients present with hyperleptinaemia (high leptin levels), but this has been interpreted as evidence of leptin resistance, suggesting a reduced sensitivity to leptin's physiological effects.

Explanations for high concentrations of leptin in obese individuals include: a compensatory response to the absence of functional receptors as well as reduced leptin bioactivity or signalling (Frühbeck *et al.* 1998); supraphysiological leptin concentrations do not trigger maximal effects due to saturation of receptors (Yu *et al.*, 1997); or that functional leptin receptors themselves are lacking (Caro *et al.*, 1996). Additionally, there is some evidence that transport of leptin receptor isoforms may be abnormal in obesity (Halaas JL, *et al.*, 1997) or that there might be a decreased capacity (Caro *et al.*, 1996; Banks et al., 1996) of leptin transport in cerebrospinal fluid.

In preliminary trials of a candidate drug, 165 subjects were randomised to receive either leptin or placebo, in addition to exercise and nutrition counselling. For all subjects who completed at least 28 days of the study, 19% of placebo patients lost at least 2kg and 30-45% of patients treated with doses of leptin lost at least 2kg. For the 30 obese subjects who remained in the study for 90 days, the mean weight losses were 2-4kg and 1.5kg for those receiving leptin and placebo, respectively. However, the weight reduction could also be interpreted as that due to exercise and nutrition so care should be given when interpreting any drug trial data.

Uncoupling proteins

Proteins found on the membrane of mitochondria—sites of cell respiration—have been linked to obesity (Cinti *et al.*, 1989). The uncoupling protein-1 (UCP1) is an inner mitochondrial membrane protein found in brown adipocytes (Klaus *et al.*, 1991) and is responsible for producing heat (Cannon & Nedergaard 1985). UCP1 was originally thought to be exclusively found in brown adipose tissue (BAT), but is now found to be a member of a family of uncoupling proteins expressed in humans, animals and even plants (Laloi *et al.*, 1997). Other UCPs have been found—UCP2 and UCP3—which are also expressed in humans and animals. In genetically obese rodents activity of brown adipose tissue is reduced and the level of UCP1 mRNA and/or UCP1 is lowered (Ricquier *et al.*, 1986).

Scientists have suggested that these uncoupling proteins might play a role in energy balance and weight gain in humans. Mutations in their genes could be predictors of obesity or NIDDM (Boss *et al.*, 1998).

What about the food we eat?

Dietary fat

Excessive dietary fat intake is perhaps the universal evil in everyones mind as to what causes us to be overweight. It has been implicated in the cause of obesity for decades. However, this only represents one factor in the complex multifactorial nature of the condition. Weight-for-weight, fat provides more energy than carbohydrate or protein (Jones & Kitts 1994); it may contribute to obesity independently of its role in energy balance (Astrup & Raben 1992); it can influence food intake, energy metabolism, and substrate oxidation; high-fat foods are preferentially selected by individuals because of their high palatability (Rolls & Snide 1992); and it has a weak satiety effect (Rolls 1995).

A nutritional study (Alfieri *et al.* 1997) compared fat intake of normal weight, moderately obese and severely obese subjects and found that subjects in the moderately and severely obese groups consumed significantly more fat and cholesterol and less carbohydrate than did normal weight subjects. Obese participants also had higher intakes of saturated, monosaturated and polyunsaturated fat compared with normal weight subjects. A further study (Tucker & Kano 1992) reported that a positive association was found between dietary fat and adiposity after adjusting for age, total energy intake, physical activity level, and smoking status.

Recently, there has been a difference of opinion about whether the percentage of dietary fat plays an important role in the rising prevalence of overweight and in its treatment once it has developed. Obesity experts reviewed the results of 28 clinical trials that studied the effects of a reduction in the amount of energy from dietary fat. They showed that a reduction of 10% in the proportion of energy from fat was associated with a reduction in weight of 16g/d and concluded that dietary fat plays a role in the development of obesity. However, these data were criticised for being nonexperimental, short-term, and nonrepresentative of the world. It was also pointed out that the association between fat and body weight was only marginally significant and that the review failed to include the largest study of the relation between dietary fat and weight change (Knopp *et al.,* 1997). Subjects in this study were randomly assigned to one of four levels of fat intake for 1 year. Results showed that after one year there were no differences in weight change among the four groups.

Nevertheless, researchers generally conclude that a high fat diet may promote overweight and obesity independently of its calorie contribution.

Can viruses cause our overweight and obesity?

An interesting and radical concept suggests that obesity is caused by a viral infection. At least five different viruses have been shown to cause obesity in animals but only one—AD-36—was isolated in humans (Wigand *et al.*, 1980). AD-36 is an adenovirus, a family of viruses commonly associated with upper respiratory tract infections, which may cause enteritis and conjunctivitis. Data from Dr Nikhil Dhurandhar from the University of Wisconsin Medical School, USA, showed that serum samples obtained from obese subjects had a 30% prevalence of the human AD-36 virus compared with 5% for nonobese subjects. Dr Dhurandhar concluded that there is a strong association to show that human adenovirus causes overweight and obesity although the exact mechanism is unknown and that further investigations are needed.

For ethical reasons, experimental viral inoculation in humans cannot be performed therefore most studies will be required to focus on the indirect evidence of AD-36 in already infected obese humans.

What about our external stimuli such as our environment—do these have a part to play in being overweight?

Physical activity and exercise

Physical activity plays an important role in weight loss and weight gain. Physically active individuals have been shown to be less likely to gain weight; they are more likely to produce lean mass; and they have increased metabolic benefits with respect to blood lipid composition. However, studies have failed to show an association between physical activity and weight gain (Williamson *et al.*, 1993; Klesges *et al.*, 1992), but these have been criticised as flawed because of confounding physical activity level (PAL) assessment tools, such as the use of one measurement of physical activity instead of multiple measurements.

One study (Rippe & Hess, 1998) has consoliodated the views of others by explaining the relationship between physical activity and obesity. It concludes that:

- The combination of physical activity and dietary restriction is more effective for weight loss than dietary restriction alone
- Physical activity affects body composition favourably during weight loss by increasing or preserving fat-free mass
- Physical activity affects the rate of weight loss in a dose-response manner which is based on both the frequency and duration of physical activity

Additionally, physical activity may also affect the distribution of body fat. Studies have shown an inverse relationship between levels of physical activity and indirect measures of body fat distribution (eg WHR) (Seidell *et al.*, 1991; Tremblay *et al.*, 1990). Other population-based studies (Seidell *et al.*, 1991; Troisi *et al.*, 1991) have shown that active men and women have lower WHRs than their sedentary counterparts.

Other studies have shown that exercise enhances body image, boosts self-esteem, and improves mood (Brownell 1995).

Physically inactive individuals might also be predisposed to not engaging in physical activities because of muscle fibre types and metabolic characteristics: obesity-prone rats (Mrad *et al* 1992) and obese persons (Wade *et al.*, 1990) have an increased proportion of fast-twitch muscle fibres, which have decreased oxidative capacity (Pette & Spamer 1986) and oxidize less lipid during steady-state exercise (Wade *et al.*, 1990). Differences in the muscle oxidative capacity may influence the perceived level of fatigue and, hence, the capacity or tendency to be physically active (Weinsier *et al.*, 1998).

A randomised trial (Andersen *et al.*, 1999) of the effects of lifestyle activity versus structured aerobic exercise in overweight obese women found that after a 16-week period while on a low-fat diet, those in the aerobic exercise group lost on average 8.3 kg compared with 7.9 kg for the lifestyle activity group. Other improvements were found in systolic blood pressure and serum lipid and lipoprotein levels. This study confirmed that sedentary overweight individuals can reduce weight by adopting gradual and moderate intensity physical activity (eg. walking instead of driving, take stairs instead of escalators), which contributes to enhanced weight management and improved cardiovascular risk profiles. This study is supported by further evidence (Dunn *et al*, 1999) that behaviourally based lifestyle physical activity interventions can significantly improve cardiorespiratory fitness, blood pressure, and body composition.

In summary, physical activity may facilitate weight maintenance and weight loss through direct energy expenditure and improved physical fitness. Exercise may help to equate fat intake with fat oxidation rates thereby reducing excess fat mass—an effect most visible in professional sportsmen and women where the prevalence of obesity is almost zero.

Is it all in the mind?

Psychosocial factors

Cognitive psychology is an important aspect of human feeding. Memories and taste preferences are uniquely involved in macronutrient selection (ie, eating a chocolate bar rather than a bowl of kidney beans), satiety, and feeding frequency; and activity-related behaviours are governed by attitudes to health and fitness. Additionally, the obesity epidemic is viewed by some to be caused by modern day psychosocial and lifestyle influences such as the 'comfort' eating of foods during times of emotional stress; the ingestion of large quantities of high fat, high carbohydrate foods at regular family gatherings; the 'silent' consumption or 'snacking' of fatty foods during long periods of inactivity such as watching television or sitting in an office.

Psychological distress—including poor mood, depression, and low self-esteem—may also exacerbate overeating, and obesity may result from difficult life events such as abuse, addiction, or marital or family dysfunction. Psychology has provided a few theories to explain obesity and weight gain and although they pose interesting areas of causation, the role of psychosocial factors in obesity is only one piece of the complicated puzzle of why we gain weight.

Let us look at some interesting areas where psychology takes a role in eating behaviour.

Appetite control

Laboratory studies on overweight/obese people showed that following a covert energy preload (unknown infusion of high energy foods) obese subjects had a reduced capacity to accurately compensate for the energy content of the pre-load at a subsequent meal compared with lean subjects resulting in overeating and increased energy intake (Spiegal *et al.*, 1989). This suggests that obese individuals are unable to control their appetite adequately.

Taste preference

Psychological studies suggest that the perception of palatability might influence the amount and type of food consumed. Dietary fat has been shown to exhibit weak satiating properties and subjects readily overeat in response to high fat foods (Lawton *et al.*, 1993; Blundell *et al.*, 1995). Another study showed that obese women expressed a preference for fat, whereas anorectic, low BMI women expressed a preference for high sugar content foods (Drewnowski *et al.*, 1987).

External cues

Evidence that eating behaviour in overweight/obese individuals appeared to be more sensitive to external cues such as the time of day, sight or smell of food or the presence of others first came from Schacter in 1971. For example, obese people eat more than normal weight people when food tastes good but eat less than normal weight individuals when it tastes bad. This increased responsiveness to food cues suggests that overweight individuals may be more susceptible to overindulging during meal times. One study showed that obese diners were more influenced by the description or display of a dessert than nonobese diners (Herman *et al.*, 1983). This 'externality theory' has been shown to correlate with BMI (Strien *et al.*, 1995) and more recently has been shown to be associated with greater consumption of preferred foods (Spitzer and Rodin 1981).

Eating disorders

A number of psychological disorders have been associated with obesity. Binge eating occurs when individuals consume large amounts of food with the subjective sensation of loss of control. Researchers have linked binge eating to the onset of obesity whereas others have linked it to emotional distress (Mussell *et al.*, 1995). Although there is evidence of a higher level of personality disorders and depression in binge eaters, most cases report that the eating disorder precedes the development of other comorbidity (Jebb 1997).

Stress

There is some evidence that emotional stress might play a role in the progression of weight gain and obesity. Stress has been linked to overconsumption of high fat foods and a community based study showed that weight gain was associated with stress (McGann *et al.*, 1990). A further study proposed that abdominal obesity was caused by stress through brain pathways (Bjorntorp 1993).

Environmental and sociocultural factors

Perhaps the most striking examples of the effects of the environment on obesity come from studies on the Naura in Micronesia, and Polynesians in Western Samoa. Because of dramatic changes in diet and lifestyle in these populations over a short period, obesity prevalence has increased to 60% or more (James 1996). Genetic migrant studies have also shown that different environmental circumstances can alter average weight by as much as 25kg (Ravussin 1995). A study showed that migrant Africans living in the Caribbean or US showed a significant increase in the prevalence of obesity compared with their native countries of Nigeria or Cameroon (Wilks *et al.*, 1996).

Cross-cultural studies of physical activity and BMI have reported a sevenfold increased risk of being overweight and within developed countries there is a relationship between low levels of physical activity and an increased risk of becoming obese (Ferro-Luzzi & Martino L, 1996).

Another environmental factor associated with obesity includes the sedentary behaviours of TV viewing (Gortmaker *et al.*,1996).

Socioeconomic studies show a strong class gradient with regard to the cause of obesity (Bennett *et al.*,1995; Jebb *et al.*, 1997). Analysis suggest that in the UK, the prevalence of obesity among women ranges from 10.7% in high social classes compared with 25% in the lower social classes. This effect might, however, be due to the types of food consumed, quantity of food consumed, education about food content, physical activity, and affordability of food.

Other sociocultural factors that are associated with obesity include gender, ethnicity, familial hierarchies, and social and moral pressures, but their true contribution in the aetiology of obesity remain to be elucidated.

CHAPTER 3

Health Risks of Fat

There are many health risks associated with fatness. Excess body mass increases the risk of death from the following disorders: heart disease or cardiovascular diseases (CVD), non-insulin dependent diabetes mellitus (NIDDM), hypertension, respiratory disorders, gallbladder disease, and certain cancers (Lee 1993; Pi-Sunyer 1993). The health consequences of obesity are varied, ranging from sudden death (Bray 1992) to several chronic complaints that diminish an individual's quality of life.

It has been shown that the location as well as volume of body fat can determine health risks (Després 1993). Patients with intra-abdominal or android obesity tend to develop insulin-resistance syndrome, hyperinsulinaemia, dyslipidaemia (abnormal fat concentrations in the blood), and hypertension (Després 1993; Després 1994). Additionally, these studies have shown a correlation between android obesity and increased risk for coronary artery disease, stroke, diabetes mellitus, and mortality.

Cardiovascular Disease (CVD)

Being overweight and obese increases the risk of CVD in both men and women (Hubert *et al.*, 1983). Essential hypertension, left ventricular hypertrophy, arrhythmias, stroke, myocardial infarction, angina pectoris, congestive heart failure, and peripheral vascular disease have all been identified as cardiovascular risk factors in obese patients. Mortality rates due to CVD are almost 50% higher in obese individuals compared with those of average weight, and as high as 90% in those with severe obesity (Alpert & Hashimi 1993). The National Institute of Diabetes and Digestive and Kidney Diseases (NIDDKD) Statistics in the US report that nearly 70% of diagnosed cases of cardiovascular disease are related to obesity.

Hypertension (High Blood Pressure)

Hypertension has been reported in 66% of overweight/obese patients (Zemel 1995). Researchers have suggested that hyperinsulinaemia might cause renal sodium retention and associated blood pressure increases via stimulation of the sympathetic nervous system (Alpert *et al.*, 1994). The US National Health and Nutrition Examination Survey II (NHANES II) survey showed that the prevalence of hypertension in overweight adults is 2.9-fold higher than that observed in normal weight adults (Van Itallie 1985). The risk of hypertension increases with the duration of obesity, however weight reduction reduces this risk, especially in women (Huang *et al.*, 1998).

Stroke

The Honolulu study (Abbott *et al.*, 1994) found that elevated BMI was associated with risk of thromboembolic stroke and other studies (Larsson *et al.*, 1984; Lapidus *et al.*, 1984) have found similar anthropometric associations. However, data from women in the Swedish Obese Subjects (SOS) study were inconclusive (Sjöström 1992).

Dyslipidaemia (Abnormal Lipid Levels)

Obese individuals, especially those with visceral obesity ('apple' shaped), are frequently characterised by a dyslipidaemic state that exacerbates a genetic predisposition to coronary artery disease (Després 1994). Generally, the lipid profile of obese individuals shows raised plasma triglyceride levels, raised low-density lipoprotein-apolipoprotein B (LDL-apoB) levels, and reduced high-density lipoprotein-cholesterol (HDL-C) levels (Després 1990).

Cardiomyopathy (Heart Defects)

Cardiac defects have been identied more commonly in long-term obese patients compared with those who have had obesity for a shorter period: fatty infiltration of the myocardium, right ventricular hypertrophy, excess epicardial fat, abnormalities of ventricular function, and increased left ventricular filling pressure appear to be closely related to the duration of obesity (Hubert *et al.*, 1983; Thompson 1997).

Non-insulin-dependent diabetes mellitus (NIDDM)

There is a strong association between obesity and the risk of developing NIDDM (Skarfors et al., 1991; McKeigue et al., 1992; Cassano et al.,1992). The risk of NIDDM increases continuously with BMI and decreases with weight reduction: data suggests that approximately 64% of obese men and 74% of obese women could have prevented NIDDM if their BMI was below 25 (Chan et al., 1994). The 1998 NIDDKD statistics report that nearly 80% of patients with NIDDM are obese.

Certain characteristics of obese individuals have been found to predispose them to NIDDM after controlling for age, smoking, and familial inheritance of the disorder. These include childhood and adolescent obesity, intra-abdominal fat mass accumulation, and progressive weight gain from eighteen years of age onwards (Chou et al.; 1994; Lundgren et al., 1989).

It is thought that as weight is gained, an increased demand for insulin possibly leads to insulin resistance and hyperinsulinemia and, ultimately, NIDDM (Després 1993). Metabolic abnormalities may also promote insulin resistance: obese patients tend to have increased plasma free fatty acid levels, which may interfere with insulin sensitivity in the muscles; and accumulation of fat in the intra-abdominal tissues might lead to high portal vein concentrations of free fatty acids, which may in turn inhibit hepatic clearance of portal insulin (Bjorntorp 1995).

Additionally, steroid hormone abnormalities such as hypercortisolaemia and hyperandrogenicity, which play an important role in the regulation of insulin sensitivity in muscle tissue and liver (Bjorntorp 1995), might contribute to the progression of NIDDM. Physical and chronic psychological stress may also exacerbate insulin resistance or NIDDM (Bjorntorp 1995).

Risk factors for NIDDM include a high waist-to-hip ratio (android obesity), large waist circumference (visceral adiposity), overall obesity, insulin resistance, dyslipidaemia (hypertriglyceridaemia and hypercholesterolemia, increased LDL-C, decreased HDL-C), lack of physical activity, and gestational diabetes mellitus (Haffner 1995).

From cross-cultural studies, obesity and NIDDM is especially prevalent among African-Americans, Hispanic Americans, and American Indians (Raymond & D'Eramo-Melkus 1993).

Insulin resistance

The metabolic syndrome, also known as Syndrome X or the Insulin Resistance Syndrome, is another disorder associated with abnormal lipid profiles and obesity. Insulin resistance and hyperinsulinaemia have been proposed as the causes linking several components of the syndrome (Ferrannini *et al.*, 1991) and diagnosis is based on two or more of the following:

- Impaired glucose tolerance
- Elevated blood pressure
- Hypertriglyceridaemia and low HDL-C
- Insulin resistance
- Central obesity

Respiratory Disease

Respiratory function and lung structure are impaired in overweight/obese individuals mainly as a result of the rigidity of the thoracic cage—caused by the accumulation of adipose tissue in and around the rib cage, abdomen and diaphragm (Nairnark & Cherniack 1960). Hypoxaemia is common (Holley et al., 1967) and sleep apnoea occurs in more than 10% of men and women with a BMI of 30 or above (Vgontzas *et al.*, 1994; Strollo & Rogers 1996). Obstructive sleep apnoea is related to central obesity and more specifically neck size—the weight of the neck on the upper airway causing narrowing when lying down. Disruption of sleep is associated with daytime somnolence, hypercapnia, morning headaches, pulmonary hypertension and, eventually, right ventricular failure (Vgontzas *et al.*, 1994; Strollo & Rogers 1996).
Most patients with sleep apnea are men, and androgens may also have a role in the pathogenesis of this syndrome (Douglas 1995).

In severe cases, obesity-hypoventilation syndrome (pickwickian syndrome) and cor pulmonale can occur and is frequently fatal (Pi-Sunyer 1993).

Gallbladder Disease

Generally speaking, gallstones occur more commonly in women and the eld-erly. However, they occur three to four times more often in obese individuals compared with nonobese individuals and is greater with central adiposity. The relative risk increases with body mass index and data suggest that being mod-erately overweight might increase the risk (Maclure *et al.,* 1989).

The underlying factors of gallstone formation in obese individuals are thought to be caused by supersaturation of bile and reduced motility of the gallbladder. Acute and chronic cholecystitis, biliary colic, and pancreatitis are other poten-tial complications from gallstones.

Interestingly, dieting and rapid weight loss also increase the risk of occurrence of gallstones (Yang *et al.,* 1992; Everhart 1993).

Cancer

Scientific studies have found a positive association between certain forms of cancer and being overweight. Obese women tend to have an increased mortal-ity rate from cancer of the gallbladder, biliary passages, breast (post-menopausally), uterus (cervix and endometrium), and ovaries (Garfinkel 1985; Lew & Garfinkel 1979) compared with normal-weight women. Obese men, however, tend to have higher rate of mortality from rectal and prostate cancer than normal-weight men (Garfinkel 1985; Lew & Garfinkel 1979); both obese men and women have an increased risk of colon cancer.

Cancers associated with the endometrium, ovary, breast, cervix and prostate in obese individuals are thought to be caused hormonally, whereas cancers of the colon, rectum, gallbladder, pancreas, liver and kidney are thought to result from gastrointestinal and hepatic abnormalities.

Endometrial cancer

Endometrial cancer is positively associated with obesity and the risk of endometrial cancer increases up to 20-fold in the most obese women (Kissebah *et al.,* 1989). The American Cancer Society prospective study, showed that women with a BMI greater than 35 had more than a fourfold increase in mortality (Lew & Garfinkel 1979).

Breast cancer

Breast cancer is associated more commonly in obese postmenopausal women, which might be partly due to production of oestrogen in adipose tissue (Young *et al.,* 1996). Breast cancer, however, is complex and genetic factors, reproductive history, insulin, and nutritional factors may all contribute (Kuller LH). A reduced risk of breast cancer might be possible in women who avoid weight gain during adulthood, especially those who do not use postmenopausal hormones (Huang *et al.,* 1997).

Prostate Cancer

Obese men with a BMI greater than 31 have a 20-30% increase in prostate cancer-related mortality (Lew & Garfinkel 1979).

Colon cancer

There is an increased risk of mortality from cancer of the colon in both men and women with a BMI greater than 35 (Lew & Garfinkel 1979). Colon cancer has been linked to diet, including high-fat and low-fibre intake, although the associations are unclear (Steinbach et al., 1994). Distinguishing between the effects of diet and obesity is difficult because the degree of obesity might influence some cancers rather than the composition of the diet.

Reproductive dysfunction

Endocrine changes associated with being overweight/obese have a detrimental effect on female reproductive function (Pasquali & Casimirri 1993). As a consequence of hyperinsulinaemia and hyperandrogenism, women can often experience hirsutism, anovulatory cycles, amenorrhoea, decreased fertility, early menarche, and delayed menopause (Peeke & Chrousos 1995; Villa *et al.,* 1997). Such disorders are more pronounced in women with central obesity (Kopelman 1994) and are more prevalent in women with greater degrees of obesity (Hartz *et al.,* 1979).

Other obesity-related conditions

Cross-sectional studies have also identified other obesity-related conditions, which are listed in Table 1.6.

Table 1.6: Conditions associated with obesity

Presenting co-morbidity
Osteoarthritis
Gout
Oedema
Gastroesophageal reflux
Urinary stress incontinence
Idiopathic intracranial hypertension
Venous stasis disease (lower extremities)
Acanthosis nigricans
Fragilitas cutis inguinalis
Hepatic steatosis
Impaired cell-mediated immunity
Blount's disease
Pseudotumour cerebri
Obstetric complications:
Toxaemia,
Hypertension,
Increased frequency of cesarean section,
And longer labour
Psychological complications:
Depression
Low self-esteem
Emotional distress

CHAPTER 4

Are We Alone in our Fight Against Fatness?

We know from the media that the obesity epidemic is now firmly established in the developed world. Its incidence is increasing at an alarming rate and the medical community agree that urgent steps need to be taken now to stem further spread of the condition.

This chapter looks at the growing global prevalence of overweight and obesity.

Prevalence

Interestingly, being overweight or obese is more prevalent in developed countries where larger quantities of high-fat and high carbohydrate rich foods are produced, but rates vary according to sociocultural and socioeconomic influences. Demographic and cross-sectional studies have shown comparative trends in obesity, and prevalence rates, for example, have been shown to be as high as 32% in Brazil and as low as 7% in France (Saw & Rajan 1997).

In the United Kingdom, the proportion of the population who are obese tripled from 1980 to the present date and has become one of the fastest growing obesity rates in the world. In 1998, figures revealed that 19% of men and 21% of women were obese in the UK and obesity accounted for 18 million days of sickness absence and 30,000 premature deaths. Today, according to the WHO, more than 1 billion adults are overweight with at least 300 million of them clinically obese. Current obesity levels range from below 5% in China, Japan and some African nations, to over 75% in urban Samoa.

In the USA obesity affects more than 70 million people, which relates to more than 30% of the adult population and 20% of children. Prevalence rates are found to be rising consistently over many years in both sexes and especially more prevalent in non-White women (eg African-American or Mexican-American women).

Furthermore, childhood obesity is already an epidemic in some countries and on the increase in others. An estimated 22 million children under five are estimated to be overweight worldwide. According to the US Surgeon General, in the USA the number of overweight children has doubled and the number of overweight adolescents has trebled since 1980. The problem is global and increasingly extends into the developing world; for example, in Thailand the prevalence of obesity in 5-to-12 year olds children rose from12.2% to 15-16% in just two years.

CHAPTER 5

What are the Options?

The quest to find the miracle cure for eliminating fat is well and truly in full force. Pharmaceutical and supplement manufacturers are actively researching new pills and potions that promise to eliminate the fat that has accumulated within people's bodies throughout the years of consistent food intake—in addition to the prospect of lucrative commercialisation where they will strive to line their pockets with millions of dollars from blockbuster treatments.

Over the past decade there have been constant diets, books, and work-out videos that make claims to help shed pounds and these fads fuel the cycle of obsession with the body beautiful. There have been many successes and some failures along the way. Take for instance the latest diet crazes, from the GI Diet, The South Beach Diet, and the Dr Atkins diet, which all offer a different perspective to dieting based on nutrition. For example, the GI diet makes you aware of glycaemic indices of food such as how much sugar is in them, whereas the Atkins Diet suggests that people should eat more high protein, high fat foods and limited carbohydrates. Of course, these diets and plans will work for some but they may not work for others. This is because, as explained in the previous chapters, body weight regulation is not simply about nutrition and diet. It has to do with physical activity and the internal mechanisms of body weight regulation in addition to psychosocial factors.

The failures in the search for the holy grail of eliminating fat include the numerous work-out videos, medical therapies, supplements, surgery and behaviour modification.

Drugs

Antiobesity drugs have had a difficult time evolving over the years. Early use of thyroid extract in the late 1800s to achieve a desired weight produced some measure of hyperthyroidism with catabolic consequences on bone and muscle; dinitrophenol used first in 1933 produced neuropathy and cataracts (leading to its withdrawal); and the introduction of amphetamines in 1937 was followed by reports of addiction (Bray 1998).

Administration of drugs such as digitalis and diuretics (and those containing amphetamine-based preparations) led to several deaths in 1967 and prompted the US Senate to intervene; aminorex was withdrawn from the market in Europe in 1971 after links to an outbreak of pulmonary hypertension (Bray 1976); and 17 deaths occurred in 1978 which were associated with very low energy diets containing collagen as the principal source of protein (Sours *et al.*, 1981).

Longer-term treatments like dexfenfluramine and fenfluramine were withdrawn from the market because of their association with cardiac valve abnormalities.

Supplements

There are also many nutritional supplements and other diets that have been marketed for people who are overweight and obese. They range from special short-term liquid diets, low calorie food supplements to very low calorie diets. The simplest short-term liquid diet is milk, which can produce good results in those who are having difficulty in initiating weight loss. It is not recommended in the long term and can cause diarrhoea in some patients. Other liquid diets are not recommended because they are generally high in protein and are not nutritionally balanced or monitored by a physician.

There are abundant numbers of foodstuffs marketed as low calorie, fat-free, or having weight-reducing properties. Most claim to help reduce overweight but there are no long-term clinical data available to show efficacy and, at best, show only modest benefits.

Very low calorie diets (VLCD) produce early and substantial weight loss and include appropriate vitamin and mineral supplementation. They are restricted to those who have a BMI > 30 and should only be initiated after a thorough medical examination, in conjunction with a regular monitoring and a lifestyle programme. VLCD produce weight loss between 15 and 25 kg over a 3-month period but intensive management is required to maintain weight loss after the dieting programme.

Buling agents such as methylcellulose, carboxymethycellulose, psyllium hydrophilic colloid, polycarbophil, and natural fibres (eg oat bran, wheat) can produce a temporary satiating effect and can reduce the desire to eat for up to 30 minutes. However, they increase the risk of peristalsis and require large quantities of water.

Chromium is an essential trace mineral that is sold widely as a supplement believed to promote weight loss, increase muscle mass and protect against heart disease, osteoporosis and may even increase life span. Chromium became popular in 1987 after researchers (Campbell *et al.*, 1987) found that levels of chromium in blood and urine were raised after exercising.

Studies (Evans 1982; Evans 1989) using chromium picolinate supplementation over a 6-week period showed significantly higher increases in muscle mass and a greater loss of body fat than the placebo group. However, other studies have failed to reach similar conclusions (Lukaski *et al.*, 1996; Clancy *et al.*, 1994). Daily chromium supplementation was shown to significantly enhance the action of insulin (Cefalu *et al.*, 1997) in 29 overweight subjects with a family history of diabetes. Additionally, abdominal fat associated with hypertension and insulin resistance was increased by only 1% in the chromium group versus 6.5% in the placebo group although the researchers concluded that the differences in abdominal fat were not statistically significant.

Other interesting, less publicised supplements include bee products and herbal remedies. A study (Mincheva *et al.*, 1998) investigating the potential of bee products as antiobesity agents was published in the proceedings of the International Congress on Obesity, 1998. After treating 68 individuals with a hypocaloric diet enriched with bee products (propolis, bee pollen and royal jelly) a reduction of 5.76 kg was established as well as an improvement of the lean body mass/fat tissue mass ratio. Total cholesterol decreased with an average of 25.3% and the level of triglycerides dropped by 49.7%. The role of bee products in the treatment of obesity and the metabolic syndrome, as well as for the early prevention of atherosclerosis is emphasised.

Natural herbal-based products are also available to those who are overweight and readily available over the counter in chemists or pharmacies. These products also make claims of effective weight reduction but often long-term clinical trials are not conducted and their use is limited, if any benefit is discerned at all.

Surgery

A radical option to excessive overweight is surgery. This specialism, called bariatric surgery, is only offered to morbidly obese individuals with a Body Mass Index greater than 35 with life-threatening or comorbid conditions such as NIDDM, hypertension, dyslipidaemia or cardiovascular diseases. There are two main surgical options available for the treatment of severe obesity: (1) restrictive operations such as vertical banded gastroplasty, gastric stapling, or laparoscopic gastric banding; and (2) gastric bypass operations (eg Roux-en-Y gastric bypass procedure or biliopancreatic diversion). Other surgical options might include jaw wiring, intestinal bypass, and liposuction.

Gastric surgical procedures can induce rapid and substantial weight reduction within 1 year of the operation (Sugerman *et al.*, 1992) and long-term weight loss can be impressive. However, surgery should not be performed lightly owing to possible serious complications: the patient is required to make substantial lifestyle and dietary changes and must be committed to adhering to postoperative medical protocols.

Behavioural therapy

Lifestyle programs that include cognitive-behavioural techniques for dietary modification, encouragement for physical activity and support for psychological functioning are effective in facilitating short-term weight losses. Long-term success is placed on the patient's determination and commitment to adhere to behavioural modification programs, and failure to do so is the reason why many weight loss programs are ineffective in the long term.

Maintaining weight loss is perhaps more difficult than losing it initially. Therefore, relapse prevention is a major goal for most behavioural interventions (Brownell *et al.*, 1986; Marlatt & Gordon 1985). For those embarking on behavioural means of weight reduction, the social challenges of eating in groups and family gatherings, eating as a means to cope with daily stressors, and the selective eating of certain low calorie foods, in addition to physical exercise regimens makes life extremely difficult.

Counselling is also important to support and reinforce the behavioural intervention: it is important for the individual to learn that even moderate weight loss is a success and that losing 5-10% of body weight is beneficial—a perception of failure can lead to depression and weight regain (Brownell 1998).

Most psychosocial interventions last approximately 20 weeks and in the short-term induce average weight losses of 8.4 kg; however, patients maintain, on average, two-thirds of their initial weight loss 9-10 months after treatment termination. In most studies, patients tend to return to baseline within a few years after treatment termination, unless sustained psychological intervention is implemented (Perri & Fuller 1995; Safer 1991).

CHAPTER 6

The High Activity Low Obesity Plan

By now, you will have a fairly good idea that weight gain is not simply a process of dietary excess. It is a more complex balance of energy intake versus expenditure combined with the factors that drive us to eat, together with the degree to which we are physically activity. To take these various evidence-based aspects into account, the HALO Plan has been developed as a holistic lifestyle plan, which is intended to educate the overweight and normal weight about eating, the importance of physical activity in weight reduction, and the psychological components that make us eat and motivate us to become physically active. Above all else, it is intended to make our bodies healthier by reducing fat deposition.

It will use the information in the previous chapters to illustrate that weight reduction and weight management can be successfully achieved by making lifestyle changes combined with dietary advice and behaviour modification.

The plan may not suit everyone but those who are overweight or those of normal weight can use the principles to regulate their body weight. There are also useful practical tips and guidance on what types of food should be preferred and the times that food should be consumed.

Preparation for the plan

It is important to assess your health and how much change you want to make to your lifestyle. Therefore you may wish to get a check up from your GP to test blood pressure, cholesterol levels and discuss any worries or concerns that you may have in connection with starting a new lifestyle regime that involves dieting and exercise. You may also wish to sit down and create a checklist of all your current available time and how much time you can dedicate to, for example, exercise or physical activity. It is recommended that you try to dedicate at least one hour per day to some form of exercise whether that is in the form of riding a bicycle, to walking briskly, working out in the gym, swimming, or even energetic sexual activity.

Once you are happy that you have the time, resources, and motivation to embark on a new plan then you then you can embark on the Three Step Plan by first creating a food chart. This chart is required to help you understand what and how much you consume each day and week.

Step 1. The Food Chart

Make a diary of how much food and drink you consume each day for 1 week. This must include everything that you eat. This chart is important because it will make you think about what types of food you eat and the volume of food that you eat. Make a note also of the times you are eating. If you are snacking between meals put the time down that you had a snack or a drink.

Each entry is an indicator of how much you consume. For example, if you have three meals (3 x main meals, and 2 x desserts) a day plus 4 coffees and three snacks, this would amount to 12 units. In the HALO Plan it is recommended that for weight reduction and management, you limit your intake per day to no more than 9 units per day or less depending on motivational circumstances. Water can be consumed freely with no restriction and it is recommended that at least 6-8 glasses of water are consumed each day.

The food chart will also tell you the quality of the foods that you are eating. By listing the meals and their contents, you will see the percentages of carbohydrate (eg breads, pasta, rice), fats (eg. butter, milk, cream, sweets, chocolates, cakes, crisps) and protein (e.g meat, fish, eggs) that are consumed. In the HALO Plan, it is advised that only 1 unit of fat is consumed per day (ie. butter on bread, or one biscuit), but that the rest is made up of protein based foods and carbohydrates. For example, you may wish to consume three meals per day such as the following:

Breakfast   —   1 Glass of fruit juice
                         1 Banana

Lunch   — 1 Tuna pasta salad
                   1 Apple

Dinner   — 1 Chicken and rice meal
                   1 Strawberry Cheescake

Drinks   — 3-6 glasses of water
                 — 1 glass of wine
                 — 1 tea/coffee

The following pages will outline a plan for 1 month which can be repeated for three months duration. It is important to remember that this plan is flexible. For example, if more rapid weight reduction is required, then reducing the unit intake volume is an good option (eg, not a full plate of food, possibly one-half or one-third) or alternatively cutting out one of the meal times such as breakfast or lunch and substituting with a glass of fruit juice or soup. The point to this dietary plan is that the volume of food should be reduced and monitored and that the levels of exercise should be increased so that more energy is burnt off and expended. Those who wish to maintain weight should keep to a healthy eating approach and consume healthy portions and options at least twice a day and snack on only fresh fruit or vegetable type foods such as bananas, strawberries, or grapes. These foods will provide a steady level of energy without creating hunger pangs. All fast food such as pizzas, fried foods, and takeaways and high sugar fizzy drinks should *not* be consumed whilst on the diet!

Step 2. The Exercise Chart

The exercise chart should be a daily account of your physical activity. This can be the time taken to walk to the shops, to the time you worked out at home or at the gym or the bedroom workout! The time dedicated to physical activity per day is recommended at 30 minutes minimum to 1 hour. The more exercise the better but it should be done with due consideration of your health. If for example you are feeling tired or achy then a vigorous session may not be the best activity. Instead a brisk walk or a swimming session may be better. The activity should normally be vigorous and you should be perspiring at the end of the session. **If you do not perspire you are not expending enough energy to adequately burn off excess fat.**

The exercise should be viewed as fun and not a chore. Doing activity sessions in groups or classes is recommended for those with little motivation. The old adage of no pain no gain is true in the case of weight reduction. Once you get into the routine of doing physical activity it will become less of a chore and you will find that you will do it on auto-pilot. Also remember that it has probably taken years for you to lay down the fat within your body tissues through overeating and not doing exercise, so you must be prepared to persevere with the HALO Plan, as it may take years or longer to achieve your desired weight goal.

It is recommended that you are motivated each week by 'treats' that are not in an oral gratification form! These can be a visit to a hair salon, massage therapist, a leisure centre, or simply an afternoon reading a book or watching a movie. **The treats should NOT focus on food!** The more you motivate yourself to do more physical activity the more you will benefit. But remember, it may take a while to get used to increasing your physical activity but perseverance and diligence will pay off.

Step 3. The Wellbeing Chart

Your mental wellbeing is also extremely important in any weight reduction programme. If you are not focused on the eating behaviours because you are distracted then you will relapse to old habits and the dieting will not work and you will avoid exercise. This is one of the classic mistakes when people embark on faddy diets. Weight is lost initially and heralded as a success, but then the momentum is lost and weight is regained, with often more weight gained than the starting weight. Distractions may be anxieties, tensions, depression, worries, and relationship problems that may exacerbate the need to 'comfort eat'.

A wellbeing chart is best done in privacy or in a code. Write down each day how you feel about your day and how stressed, worried or anxious you are. You can use a scale of 1 to 10 to assess how you feel on a scale. If, for example, you are feeling very anxious, stressed or worried then you should rank this as a 9 or 10 whereas if you are not particularly stressed make it a 2 or 3. You must make a concerted effort to think positively even when you are experiencing low periods (when you have high scores) as these are the days when you will not adhere to the diets and the exercise regime. For the most part, you should be aiming to score low on the chart because the more exercise you do, and the healthier you become, the more the 'feel good' factor should be experienced, helping you to stick to the diet.

Motivation to stick to the HALO Plan is crucial. Rally friends round to help support you in the regime and stop you from straying into bad habits of eating wrong foods and not doing exercise. Remember your body is over 90% liquid and it needs to be looked after and kept working. The analogy here is the car engine. If you put the wrong petrol into an engine it will not work effectively and may eventually seize up. The same is true for our bodies, the more high fat, high sugar, and high protein loads you put into them, they will not work as effectively because the compounds will build up in the body causing imbalances in metabolism, storage and excretion.

CHAPTER 7

The Routine

Starting the Plan

Once you have created the Food, Exercise and Wellbeing charts, you can start the HALO Plan.

Let's look at the following four weeks and map out the daily food intake and the exercise and motivational routines.

What are the types of foods I should eat on the HALO Plan?

Fruits and vegetables	Carbohydrate	Protein	Fat
All fruits and vegetables. Examples: All leafy green varieties Avocados Peppers Tomatoes Cucumber Onions Bananas Apples Pears All berries such as strawberries, blackcurrents Raisins Dates	Rice: brown or white Low carb pasta Sweetcorn Muesli Beans Limited bread (1 sandwich per week) Limited cakes, sweets, chocolate, or biscuits! (only one portion every week).	Chicken Gammon Ham Sausage Bacon Turkey Pork Fish Limited red meat (1 portion per week) Nuts Eggs	Low fat Low sugar dressings Low fat margarine Low fat milk Low fat cheese Low fat yoghurt

Although the food is of a limited choice, it will enable rapid weight loss during the exercise routines. Once a satisfactory weight is achieved, you can introduce foods that you like as long as you maintain the exercise regimen. If you find weight is being put back on you need to cut out those foods that you reintroduced.

If you are used to eating at least three full meals a day with many snacks inbetween meals then you will experience hunger pangs during the first few weeks. The object of this diet is to restrict the volume of food you are taking in so that the exercise regime will start to burn off the fatty tissue. Also you need to retrain your stomach to receive smaller amounts of food and expect smaller amounts of food. This will be a gradual process but after a few weeks your body will become used to it.

A good tip is to prepare your meals in advance, so when you have limited time you can simply warm up the food without preparing it.

What type of exercises should I do on the HALO Plan?

Exercises
• Brisk walks
• Swimming
• Rowing machine
• Running (gym or parks)
• Bicycle riding
• Weight training
• Energetic sexual activity
• Aerobic work outs (group sessions)
• Personal trainer sessions
• Spinning
• Pillates
• Yoga
• Other exercise that causes perspiration

What can I do to keep psychologically motivated on the HALO Plan?

Stay positive and motivated by:

- Listening to favourite music
- Watching programmes on TV you enjoy
- Go to the cinema or theatre
- Participate in social events that you enjoy (eg parties)
- Go to the gym and socialise
- Be adventurous – walks, visits to new places
- Family outings/gatherings
- Visits to beauty or health salons
- Massage
- Aromatherapy
- Enjoying more sex
- Any activity that will boost your mood and energise you.

If you are experiencing low periods then it may be wise to either confide in a family member to help to support you or seek professional counselling services to help you to overcome your problems. Positivity about your diet and health will be extremely beneficial to self-esteem, confidence and self-image. So you need to take care of your psychological health as well as your physical health in order to fully appreciate the effects of the diet and the physical activity regime.

The Day-by-Day Routine

Week 1.

Monday

Note that if any of the foods are disliked you can substitute for those that are preferred on these menus. All menus are examples and it is recommended that you either follow the prescribed menus or mix-and-match foods itemised above to suit your preferred taste.

- Don't forget to weigh yourself before the start of the plan and after each 4 weeks!

Diet:	8-9am—Fruit Juice + banana
	10-11—Coffee or tea
	11-12—Portion of grapes
	12-1pm—Exercise
	1-2—Bowl of tuna pasta + water
	2-3—Water or coffee
	3-4—Apple
	4-5—Nothing
	5-6—Exercise
	6-7—Pan fried chicken in tomato sauce + rice (medium sized) +
	1 x dessert (eg cheesecake or fruit salad)
	9-12—Try to avoid food after 9pm.
Exercise:	At least 30 minutes of brisk walking or swimming between 12 and 1pm (or lunchtime or before work) and between 5 and 6pm or after work)
Wellbeing :	Take note of your diary and compare your food intake before and today. If hunger pangs are affecting your wellbeing then compensate by focusing on recreational activities such as watching a good movie or talking on the telephone with friends.

Week 1.

Tuesday

Diet:	8-9am—Bowl of muesli with nuts and fruits
	10-11—Coffee or tea
	11-12—Apple
	12-1pm—Exercise
	1-2—1 x brown bread sandwich (any filling) + water
	2-3—Water or coffee
	3-4—Portion of strawberries
	4-5—Nothing
	5-6—Exercise
	6-7—Poached salmon + spinach + mashed potato (medium)
	1 x dessert (eg cheesecake or fruit salad)
	9-12—Try to avoid food during this time as it will not digest properly. If you need something to stop hunger, drink a low fat, low calorie drink.
Exercise:	At least 30 minutes of activity between 12 and 1pm (or lunchtime or before work) and between 5 and 6pm or after work) Try a group activity session such as aerobics, yoga or pillates.
Wellbeing :	Take note of your diary and compare your food intake before and today. If you are eating less than your original diet then stay on the HALO diet. If you are eating more on HALO diet than your original diet then cut down your intake by removing a snacking meal or a main meal. Try to keep focused and think of something that excites you!

Week 1.

Wednesday

Diet:	8-9am—Fruit Juice + Scrambled Eggs on Brown Toast
	10-11—Coffee or tea
	11-12—Orange
	12-1pm—Exercise
	1-2—Salad Bowl + Water
	2-3—Water or coffee
	3-4—Mixed nuts/raisins (I portion)
	4-5—Nothing
	5-6—Exercise
	6-7—Tuna + sweetcorn + peppers +
	boiled egg white + low fat salad cream dressing (medium)
	1 x low fat yoghurt
	9-12—Try to avoid food during this time

Exercise:	At least 30 minutes of activity between 12 and 1pm
	(or lunchtime or before work) and between 5 and 6pm or after work)
	Walk, run or gym work out.

Wellbeing :	Take note of your diary and compare your food intake before and today. If you are eating less than your original diet then stay on the diet. If you are eating more on the HALO diet than your original diet then cut down your intake by removing a snacking meal or a main meal. The exercise may begin to tire you at this point. You need to now concentrate on getting to the end of the week and seek pleasurable experiences such as the benefits of losing excess weight.

Week 1.

Thursday

Diet:	8-9am—Banana + yoghurt
	10-11—Coffee or tea or water
	11-12—Pear
	12-1pm—Exercise
	1-2—Chicken Salad + Water
	2-3—Water or coffee
	3-4—Strawberries (1 portion)
	4-5—Nothing
	5-6—Exercise
	6-7—Gammon or Pork Steak + spinach + honey and mustard sauce
	1 x mousse dessert
	9-12—Try to avoid food during this time
Exercise:	At least 30 minutes of activity between 12 and 1pm (or lunchtime or before work) and between 5 and 6pm or after work) Do only 30 mins of exercise today.
Wellbeing :	Take note of your diary and compare your food intake before and today. If you are eating less than your original diet then stay on the HALO diet. If you are eating more on the HALO diet than your original diet then cut down your intake by removing a snacking meal or a main meal. Plan the weekend and avoid any temptation to eat more than 9 units of intake.

Week 1.

Friday

<table>
<tr><td>Diet:</td><td>8-9am—Bacon + Eggs, no toast/bread
10-11—Coffee or tea or water
11-12—Nothing
12-1pm—Exercise
1-2—Mixed salad bowl
2-3—Water or coffee
3-4—Mixed dried fruit (1 small portion)
4-5—Nothing
5-6—Exercise
6-7—Gammon steak + steamed vegetables (carrots, green beans)
9-12—Try to avoid food during this time</td></tr>
<tr><td>Exercise:</td><td>At least 30 minutes of activity between 12 and 1pm
(or lunchtime or before work) and between 5 and 6pm or after work)
Rowing machine + treadmill</td></tr>
<tr><td>Wellbeing :</td><td>Take note of your diary and compare your food intake before and today. You should be eating less than your original diet. If not then decrease the food intake. You should be in high spirits that you have nearly completed the first week of the diet. Treat yourself to an outing to celebrate! Keep positive about losing weight.</td></tr>
</table>

Week 1.

Saturday

Diet:	8-9am—Fruit Juice + Banana
	10-11—Coffee or tea or water
	11-12—Exercise
	12-1pm—Exercise
	1-2—Chicken tortilla wrap + water
	2-3—Water or coffee
	3-4—Apple
	4-5—Exercise
	5-6—Exercise
	6-7—Haddock + asparagus + carrots
	1 x carrot cake (1 medium slice)
	9-12—Try to avoid food during this time
Exercise:	At least 1 hour of activity between 11 and 1pm (or lunchtime or before work) and between 4 and 6pm Brisk running + any other activity
Wellbeing :	Take note of your diary and compare your food intake before and today. You should be eating less than your original diet. If not then decrease the food intake. You should be optimistic about losing weight. Try to gather support from other family members to keep you going through next week.

Week 1.

Sunday

<table>
<tr><td>Diet:</td><td>8-9am—Ham Omelette + Fruit Juice</td></tr>
<tr><td></td><td>10-11—Coffee or tea or water</td></tr>
<tr><td></td><td>11-12—Exercise</td></tr>
<tr><td></td><td>12-1pm—Exercise</td></tr>
<tr><td></td><td>1-2—Chicken + vegetables + potatoes</td></tr>
<tr><td></td><td>1 x yoghurt</td></tr>
<tr><td></td><td>2-3—Water or coffee</td></tr>
<tr><td></td><td>3-4—Orange</td></tr>
<tr><td></td><td>4-5—Exercise</td></tr>
<tr><td></td><td>5-6—Exercise</td></tr>
<tr><td></td><td>6-7—Soup + Ham Salad</td></tr>
<tr><td></td><td>1 x Fruit Salad Bowl</td></tr>
<tr><td></td><td>9-12—Try to avoid food during this time</td></tr>
<tr><td>Exercise:</td><td>At least 1 hour of activity between 11 and 1pm
(or lunchtime or before work) and between 4 and 6pm
Any activity</td></tr>
<tr><td>Wellbeing :</td><td>Take note of your diary and compare your food intake before and today. You should be eating less than your original diet. If not then decrease the food intake. You should be positive about moving onto Week 2. Note your weight on Sunday and compare with your starting weight. You may not lose any weight until the next few weeks so do not be disheartened. If you have lost weight, congratulations you will probably lose more next week if you stick to the plan. Don't avoid exercise!</td></tr>
</table>

Week 2.

Monday

- Don't forget to weigh yourself before week 2!

Diet:	8-9am—Fruit Juice + Banana
	10-11—Coffee or tea or water
	11-12—Nothing
	12-1pm—Exercise
	1-2—1 Bowl of Muesli + 1 yoghurt
	2-3—Water or coffee
	3-4—Orange
	4-5—Nothing
	5-6—Exercise
	6-7—1 x Pasta with bacon + cream sauce
	1 x glass wine
	9-12—Try to avoid food during this time
Exercise:	At least 1 hour of activity between 12 and 1pm (or lunchtime or before work) and between 5 and 6pm Any activity
Wellbeing :	You should be feeling the effects of exercise. If you are tired then take less exercise but restart the enthusiasm when you are less tired. You should find that the more exercise you do the more energy you have. If you are hungry then do not eat more, continue with the plan and make arrangements to visit people, socialise and go out for recreational activities. Your wellbeing scores should be average.

Week 2.

Tuesday

Diet: 8-9am—Fruit Juice + Scrambled Eggs (No toast)
                10-11—Nothing
                11-12—Small portion of grapes
            12-1pm—Exercise
                1-2—1 x Chicken Salad
                2-3—Water or coffee
                3-4—Orange
                4-5—Nothing
                5-6—Exercise
                6-7—Pork steak with steamed vegetables (medium portions)
                    0.5 Melon
                9-12—Try to avoid food during this time

Exercise: At least 1 hour of activity between 12 and 1pm
            (or lunchtime or before work) and between 5 and 6pm
            Any activity—keep to group activity if you prefer this.

Wellbeing : You should be rewarding yourself by treats such as
            soaking in the bath with no distractions, playing music,
            or watching movies. You need to make sure you can stay on
            the diet for the next three weeks so keep motivated by having
            support from your colleagues and family and friends.

Week 2.

Wednesday

Diet:	8-9am—Fruit Juice + Banana
	10-11—Nothing
	11-12—Strawberries + Grapes (1 bowl)
	12-1pm—Exercise
	1-2—1 x tortilla wrap (meat or vegetable)
	2-3—Water or coffee
	3-4—Nothing
	4-5—Nothing
	5-6—Exercise
	6-7—Pork steak with broccoli + steamed vegetables (medium portions)
	1 x yoghurt
	9-12—Try to avoid food during this time
Exercise:	At least 1 hour of activity between 12 and 1pm (or lunchtime or before work) and between 5 and 6pm Any activity—keep to group activity if you prefer this.
Wellbeing:	You may be feeling more hunger pangs as the food intake is gradually reduced. Try to stick to the plan with your will power to lose weight. Drink fruit juice if you are severely hungry or eat mints or brush your teeth when you are feeling hungry—the taste of mint after orange juice or vice versa will stem the hunger pangs for a while until you can eat a main meal. Keep focused and drink plenty of water during your exercise routines.

Week 2.

Thursday

Diet:	8-9am—Nothing
	10-11—Coffee or tea
	11-12—Banana + Grapes
	12-1pm—Exercise
	1-2—1 x brown bread sandwich (any filling)
	1 x yoghurt
	2-3—Water or coffee
	3-4—Nothing
	4-5—Nothing
	5-6—Exercise
	6-7—Chicken Tikka Masala + rice
	1 x glass wine
	9-12—Try to avoid food during this time

Exercise:	At least 1 hour of activity between 12 and 1pm (or lunchtime or before work) and between 5 and 6pm Any activity—keep to group activity if you prefer this.

Wellbeing:	You may be feeling more hunger pangs as the food intake is gradually reduced. Try to stick to the plan with your will power to lose weight. Drink fruit juice if you are severely hungry or eat mints or brush your teeth when you are feeling hungry—the taste of mint after orange juice or vice versa will stem the hunger pangs for a while until you can eat a main meal. Keep focused and drink plenty of water during your exercise routines. Rally support from friends and family.

Week 2.

Friday

Diet:	8-9am—Nothing
	10-11—Coffee or tea
	11-12—Apple + Cereal Bar
	12-1pm—Exercise
	1-2—Chicken Pasta Bowl
	2-3—Water or coffee
	3-4—Nothing
	4-5—Nothing
	5-6—Exercise
	6-7—Pork chop + steamed or boiled vegetables
	9-12—Try to avoid food during this time
Exercise:	At least 1 hour of activity between 12 and 1pm (or lunchtime or before work) and between 5 and 6pm Any activity—keep to group activity if you prefer this.
Wellbeing:	You may be feeling more hunger pangs as the food intake is gradually reduced. Try to stick to the plan with your will power to lose weight. Drink fruit juice if you are severely hungry or eat mints or brush your teeth when you are feeling hungry—the taste of mint after orange juice or vice versa will stem the hunger pangs for a while until you can eat a main meal. Keep focused and drink plenty of water during your exercise routines. Rally support from friends and family.

Week 2.

Saturday

Diet:	8-9am—Bacon + Eggs + Beans + Toast (1 piece)
	10-11—Coffee or tea or water
	11-12—Exercise
	12-1pm—Exercise
	1-2—Bowl of Muesli + Banana
	2-3—Water or coffee
	3-4—Apple
	4-5—Exercise
	5-6—Exercise
	6-7—Salmon + broccoli + carrots
	0.5 Melon
	9-12—Try to avoid food during this time
Exercise:	At least 1 hour of activity between 11 and 1pm (or lunchtime or before work) and between 4 and 6pm Any activity
Wellbeing:	If you are hungry, eat some nuts and raisins inbetween meals to stem the hunger. Keep a positive attitude that the week is nearly ended. If you are tired, slow down the exercise and relax in a bath with a glass of wine. Make plans for the weekend and enjoy the plan.

Week 2.

Sunday

Diet:	8-9am—Muesli + raisins + dried fruit
	10-11—Coffee or tea or water
	11-12—Exercise
	12-1pm—Exercise
	1-2—Gammon steak + pineapple
	2-3—Water or coffee
	3-4—Apple
	4-5—Exercise
	5-6—Exercise
	6-7—Risotto + wine
	1 x cheesecake
	9-12—Try to avoid food during this time
Exercise:	At least 1 hour of activity between 11 and 1pm (or lunchtime or before work) and between 4 and 6pm. Brisk running + any other activity. Alternatively take a partner out to play tennis, football, badminton, any other activities where you will perspire!
Wellbeing:	You should by now start to see some weight reduction because you have increased your physical activity levels and cut down the volume of food that you are eating. You should congratulate yourself and treat yourself but not with food. The next two weeks will be harder as you lower your food intake further and maintain the levels of physical activity. If at any stage you feel unwell, which should be rare, you must cease the plan until you feel you can restart it.

Weeks 3 and 4

At week 3, you should follow the same plan as week 2, but you should cut down on the food intake by at least 20%. Your body will start to utilise fat depots as an alternative fuel source. So for example, instead of a full plate of food, serve yourself 20% less than a full plate. Your exercise levels should be the same as week 2. You should be energised and eating only fruits and nuts in between meals if you need to.

If you are hungry and only think of food, then you should not starve yourself, instead, eat foods that you know will give you a burst of energy such as dried fruits or a banana. Do not relapse on high fat, high sugar foods as this will STOP any benefits that you have started and worked so hard to attain.

At week 4 follow the same as week 2 but cut down food intake by a further 5% so only allow yourself a 75% intake of food compared with week 1.

Use the motivational tips and hints in the next chapter to keep you going.

Month 2-3

At 1 Month on the Plan you should have lost weight. This is because you have worked to retrain your body to expect less food and utilise stored fat as an energy source. You are doing well. You should now set yourself a target weight and use the principles of the HALO Plan to steer you towards this goal.

Over the next two months you should not decrease food intake further because it is essential that you have daily portions of carbohydrate, protein, and fat. But you should try to increase activity levels through intensity rather than more time. For example make the work-outs harder by increasing weights or cycling faster so that you perspire more readily or spend more times a week going to group sessions such as yoga or aerobic classes. Take stairs instead of lifts and walk wherever permitting.

For months 2-3 follow the diets and activity plans of Week 4 and try to increase activity levels.

CHAPTER 8

Maintaining the plan

Like all diets and exercise routines, they are difficult to stick to for long periods of time and boredom sets in. The key to successfully reducing weight and maintaining that weight loss is the psychological motivation and determination to not relapse. All too often however, our bodies tell us that we are hungry to the extent that primitive drives or psychological 'cravings' take over and the hunt and need for food becomes too much, and for the most, this will lead to binge eating on bad foods that will only put you back further in the quest for the perfect figure.

So what can be done to stop those feelings of desperation and temptation to eat the foods we so desire? On the HALO Plan, you will see that over the weeks you are re-programming your brain and stomach to receive smaller volumes of food so that the body can utilise stored food as fuel as you increase physical activity. In a similar way to surgical banding, where the stomach space is stapled and reduced so that only tiny amounts of food are allowed to pass, the restriction of food in the HALO Plan (without the need for severe surgical intervention!) serves the same goal but uses your own willpower.

In psychological literature 'Restraint theory' tells us that if you restrain yourself or stop yourself eating 'bad' foods you are more likely to eat the wrong foods often to the extent that you eat more of the wrong foods, hence 'cheating' on the diet. This may lead to weight gain over and above the starting weight. This is perhaps why many diets do not work. Although the HALO diet does say NO to all fat foods and fizzy drinks, it tells you why you should avoid them because of this restraint mechanism in our heads. Now you have read this you are more aware of this basic mechanism so you can think differently about overcoming the urge to eat the wrong foods. It is a natural process therefore to want to eat foods that you are told that are bad for you yet taste good, but keep in mind why they are bad when consumed in excess as explained in Chapter 3. To overcome this obstacle there are a few things that can be done as set out in the next section.

CHAPTER 9

The Top Tips

Here are some tips on how to maintain the diet and exercise regime on the HALO Plan and to help resist the temptation of eating the wrong foods, particularly fast foods.

Practical Tips—Food

Think of fast foods which are high in fat and sugars as the raw material. For example, transfer the thought of eating a chocolate bar to eating a whole jar of syrup. If you eat it all you will be sick. Think of eating a piece of cake as eating a lump of lard. Think of eating a fried chicken wing as eating four tablespoons of margarine. Think of the fizzy drink as a cup of acid which may do nothing beneficial than rot your teeth and strip your stomach of its lining. These thoughts should help to make you avoid eating these foods while you can refocus on eating good foods high in nutrients and which are known to be beneficial to health.

There are numerous healthy eating recipe books. Invest in these to broaden your horizons on foods that are tasty, low in fat and sugar, and balanced to substitute for the fast foods.

Eliminate all cues for fast food and fizzy drinks by throwing out fizzy drinks and frozen fast foods!

Practical Tips—Exercising

In regards to exercising, the motivational aspects are crucial to maintaining the regime. One of the problems you will encounter on any diet is hunger or lack of energy to do anything. For those overweight, the body has for many years learnt to accept a full stomach plus other intake maybe three times a day. To reduce this intake will cause some changes as your stomach signals to your brain that the food is not coming in the volume it used to. Over time on the diet, your stomach and brain will get used to the reduction of food and you should be able to overcome the pangs. However, during the time you are experiencing hunger or no energy there are a few solutions:

- Snack occasionally on fresh fruits, vegetables or nuts and dried fruits such as apricots or low fat low carb cereal bars.
- Drink low calorie low sugar drinks, such as coffee or tea, or squash
- Eat boiled sweets or biscuits (only 1 or 2!) to give you a sugar burst before and after exercise
- Eat mints or brush your teeth to stem the hunger for a temporary period
- Try to avoid eating before 12 noon on occasions (the moment food hits the stomach it sends a signal to start the cycle of food intake for the whole day. If you delay it, you delay the hunger pangs—it is known that some religions fast for 12 hours or more with nothing than water passing their mouths).
- Exercise at the pace you are comfortable with—do not over exert yourself

Practical Tips—Psychology

- Give yourself a daily reward for sticking to the diet. Make it a recreational activity or a leisure activity. Avoid food as the focus of the reward!
- Motivate yourself to exercise by thinking that no weight will vanish if you do not exercise! Remember, if you really want to lose weight and maintain it, you need to increase physical activity!
- Always think positively about your image. Think about how you want to look and use this as your yardstick to help you to resist temptation of eating the wrong foods.
- Understand how restraint theory works. Don't eat bad foods just because you have been told not too. Don't view it as restraint but more importantly that there is a justifiable reason for doing so—that is, your health will suffer if you do eat wrong foods.
- Think ahead and plan your food intake the day before and prepare it it advance!

- Be realistic—know that it will be a long road to achieve your target weight and maintain it, but when you reach it, you can maintain it!
- Be positive and optimistic about physical exercise—make it fun by exercising in groups or as couples.
- Get support from partners, family members and colleagues.
- Resist the 'lazy brain' of trying it once and not going back. Perseverance always pays off!

CHAPTER 10

The Ultimate Goal

In our quest for weight loss and weight maintenance, there are many obstacles in the path to success. For example, the temptation to eat the 'bad' foods we love and prefer, and the feelings of denial and restraint when on diets, plus the physical tiredness one may experience through diet and exercise regimes all contribute to the potential failure of a slimming plan. The ultimate goal of any diet is to reduce the weight to a target weight but in a healthy and balanced way. This HALO Plan has been developed with scientific understanding of weight intake and maintenance to help achieve these goals and educate people about food behaviours and the reasons why we overeat. Additionally, it provides an information resource on the ill effects of being overweight and obese and why we should all try to restrict our dietary intake.

The HALO Plan is not for everyone, but it will be useful to those who are overweight and do not understand why the weight does not come off when they go on diets and exercise. Of course we have choices in the modern world and some will inevitably adopt a 'happy being fat' approach whereas others may not, particularly if being overweight has a bearing on health. Remember, there are no fat athletes and in the animal world there are rarely fat or overweight animals. This is because they are constantly active and burning up energy.

We all know it is a struggle to devote the time and patience to dieting, exercise, and motivation, but with the right support and guidelines, effective weight loss and management can be achieved and sustained through eating less, exercising more and understanding our eating behaviours.

REFERENCES

Abbott RD *et al* . Body mass index and thromboembolic stroke in nonsmoking men in older middle age. The Honolulo Heart Program. Stroke, 1994, 25, 2370-2376.

Abenhaim L, *et al*.. (International Primary Pulmonary Hypertension Study Group). Appetite-suppressant drugs and the risk of primary pulmonary hypertension. New England Journal of Medicine, 1996, 355, 609-616.

Ackroff K & Sclafani A. Effects of the lipase inhibitor orlistat on intake and preference for dietary fat in rats. American Journal of Physiology, 1996, 271, R48-54.

Alfieri M, *et al.* A comparison of fat intake of normal weight, moderately obese and severely obese subjects. Obesity Surgery, 1997, 7, 9-15.

Al-Isa AN. Prevalence of obesity among adult Kuwaitis: a cross-sectional study. International Journal of Obesity & Related Metabolic Disorders, 1995, 19, 431-433

Al-Mannai A *et al.* Obesity in Bahraini adults. Journal of the Royal Society of Health, 1996, 116, 30-40.

Al-Nuaim A *et al.* Prevalence of diabetes mellitus, obesity and hypercholesterolemia in Saudi Arabia. In Musaiger AO, Miladi SS (Eds). Diet-related non-communicable diseases in the Arab countries of the Gulf. Cairo, Food and Agriculture Organization of the United Nations, 1996, 73-81.

Alpert MA & Hashimi MW. Obesity and the heart. American Journal of Medical Science, 1993, 306, 117-123.

Anderson RA *et al.* Elevated intakes of chromium improve glucose and insulin variables in individuals with NIDDM. Diabetes, 1997, 46, 1786-1791.

Andersen RE *et al.*Effects of lifestyle activity vs structured aerobic exercise in obese women. Journal of the American Medical Association, 1999, 281, 335-340.

Anderson RA *et al.* Elevated intakes of chromium improve glucose and insulin variables in individuals with NIDDM. Diabetes, 1997, 46, 1786-1791.

Apfelbaum M, *et al.* Long-term maintenance of weight loss after a very low calorie diet: a randomised blinded trial of the efficacy and tolerability of sibutramine. American Journal of Medicine, 1999, 106, 179-184.

Arch JR, *et al.* Leptin resistance in obese humans: does it exist and what does it mean? International Journal of Obesity and Related Metabolic Disorders, 1996, 22, 1159-1163.

Arch J & Wilson S. Prospects for Beta-3 adrenoceptor agonists in the treatment of obesity and diabetes. International Journal of Obesity, 1996, 20, 191-199.

Arner P: Hunting for human obesity genes? Look in the adipose tissue! International Journal of Obesity and Related Metabolic Disorders; 2000:4:S57-62

Aronne LJ. Modern medical management of obesity: the role of pharmaceutical intervention. Journal of the American Dietetic Association, 1998, 10(Suppl 2), S23-S26.

Astrup A, et al. Impaired glucose-induced thermogenesis in skeletal muscle in obesity. The role of the sympathoadrenal system. International Journal of Obesity, 1987, 11, 51-66.

Astrup A, et al. Prognostic markers for diet-induced weight loss in obese women. International Journal of Obesity, 1995, 19, 275-278.

Astrup A, et al. The effect and safety of an ephedrine/caffeine compound compared to ephedrine, caffeine and placebo in obese subjects on an energy restricted diet. A double blind trial. International Journal of Obesity, 1992, 16, 269-277.

Astrup A et al. Sibutramine and energy balance. International Journal of Obesity and Related Metabolic Disorders, 1998, 22(Suppl 1),S30-S35.

Astrup A, et al. Pharmacological and clinical studies of ephedrine and other therrmogenic agonists. Obesity Research, 1995, (Suppl 4)537S-540S.

Astrup A & Lundsgaard C. What do pharmacological approaches to obesity management offer? Linking pharmacological mechanisms of obesity management agents to clinical practice, 1998, 106(Suppl 2), 29-34.

Ballor DL, et al. Resistance weight training during caloric restriction enhances lean body weight maintenance. American Journal of Clinical Nutrition, 1998, 47, 19-25.

Balsiger BM, et al. Surgical treatment of obesity: who is an appropriate candidate? Mayo Clinic Proceedings, 1997, 72, 551-558.

Banks WA, et al. Leptin enters the brain by a saturable system independent of insulin. Peptides, 1996, 17, 305-311.

Barlow SE, Dietz WH. Obesity evaluation and treatment: expert committee recommendations. Paediatrics, 1998, 102, 1-11.

Beales P & Kopelman P. Obesity genes. Clinical Endocrinology, 1996, 45, 373-378.

Bennett N, et al. Health Survey for England 1993. London:HMSO, 1995.

Benotti PN & Forse RA. The role of gastric surgery in the multidisciplinary management of severe obesity. American Journal of Surgery, 1995, 169, 361-367.

Berger M. Pharmacological treatment of obesity: digestion and absorption inhibitors—clinical perspective. American Journal of Clinical Nutrition, 1992, 55(Suppl 1), 318S-319S.

Berger A *et al.* Uncoupling proteins: the unravelling of obesity? Increased understanding of mechanisms may lead, in time, to better drugs.
British Medical Journal, 1998, 12, 1607-1608.

Berrios X *et al.* Distribution and prevalence of major risk factors of noncommunicable diseases in selected countries: the WHO Inter-Health Programme. Bulletin of the World Health Organization, 1997, 99-108.

Bessesen DH & Faggioni R. Recently identified peptides involved in the regulation of body weight. Seminars in Oncology, 1998, 25(Suppl 6), 28-32.

Billington CJ, *et al.* Effects of intracerebroventricular injection of neuropeptide Y on energy metabolism. American Journal of Physiology, 1991, 260, R321-327.

Björntorp P. Visceral obesity: a 'civilisation syndrome'. Obesity Research, 1993, 1, 206-222.

Björntorp P. Neuroendocrine abnormalities in human obesity. Metabolism. 1995, 44(Suppl. 2), 38-41.

Blouin RA, *et al* . Pharmacokinetic considerations in obesity. J Pharm Sci, 1999, 88, 1-7.

Blundell JE, *et al.* Serotonin, eating behavior, and fat intake. Obesity Research, 1995, 3 (Suppl 4), 471S-476S.

Blundell J, *et al.* The fat paradox: fat-induced satiety signals but overconsumption on high fat foods. International Journal of Obesity, 1995, 19, 832-835.

Blundell J. Food intake and body weight regulation. In: Regulation of Body Weight. Biological and Behavioural Mechanisms. Bouchard C & Bray G (Eds) Chichester: Wiley, 1996, 111-133.

Boss O, *et al.* The uncoupling proteins: a review. European Journal of Endocrinology, 1998, 139, 1-9.

Bray GA, *et al.* Handbook of obesity. New York: Marcel Dekker, 1997.

Bray GA. The Obese Patient.Philadelphia: WB Saunders, 1976.

Bray GA. Drug treatment of obesity: don't throw the baby out with the bath water. American Journal of Clinical Nutrition, 1998, 67, 1-4.

Bray GA. The MONA LISA Hypothesis. Most obesities known are low in sympathetic activity. In: Progress in Obesity Research. Oomura Y, Tarui S, Inoue S, Shimazu T (Eds). pp61-66. London: John Libbey & Company Ltd., 1990.

Bray GA & Popkin BM. Dietary fat intake does affect obesity!. American Journal of Clinical Nutrition, 1998, 68, 1157-1173.

Bray GA, *et al.* A double-blind randomized placebo-controlled trial of sibutramine. International Journal of Obesity and Related Metabolic Disorders, 1997, 21(Suppl 1), S25-S29.

Bray GA, *et al.* Experimental obesity: a homeostatic failure die to defective nutrient stimulation of the sympathetic nervous system . Vitam Horm, 1989, 45, 1-125.

Brolin RE, *et al.*. Long-limb gastric bypass in the superobese: a prospective randomised study. Annals of Surgery, 1992, 212, 387-395.

Brownell KD. Diet, exercise and behavioural intervention: the nonpharmacological approach. European Journal of Clinical Investigations, 1998, 28(Suppl 2), 19-22.

Brownell KD, *et al.* Understanding and preventing relapse. American Psychologist, 1986, 41, 765-782.

Brownell KD Exercise in the treatment of obesity. In: Eating Disorders and Obesity: A Comprehensive Handbook. Brownell KD & Fairburn CG (Eds). New York: Guildford, 1995, 473-478

Bucket WR, Thomas PC & Luscombe GP. The pharmacology of sibutramine hydrochloride (BTS 54 524), a new antidepressant which induces rapid noradrenergic down-regulation. Prog Neuro Psychopharmacol Biol Psychiatr, 1998, 12, 575-584.

Bultman SJ et al. Molecular characterisation of the mouse agouti locus. Cell, 1992, 71, 1195-1204.

Campfield LA et al. The OB protein (leptin) pathway—a link between adipose tissue mass and central neural networks. Hormone and Metabolic Research, 1996, 28, 619-632.

Campfield LA, *et al.* Strategies and Potential Molecular Targets for Obesity Treatment. Science, 1998, 280, 1383-1387.

Cardiac valvulopathy associated with exposure to fenfluramine or dexfenfluramine: US Department of Health and Human Services interim public health recommendations, November 1997. MMWR Morb Mortal Wkly Rep 1997, 46, 1061-1066.

Cannon B & Nedergaard J. The biochemistry of an inefficient tissue: brown adipose tissue. Essays in Biochemistry, 1985, 20, 110-164.

Caro JF, *et al.* Decreased cerebrospinal fuid/seum leptin ratio in obesity: a possible mechanism for leptin resistance. Lancet, 1996, 348, 159-161.

Carpenter WH, *et al.* Influence of body composition and resting metabolic rate on variation in total energy expenditure: a meta analysis. American Journal of Clinical Nutrition, 1995, 61, 4-10.

Carro E, *et al.* Role of Growth Hormone (GH)-Releasing Hormone and Somatostatin on Leptin-Induced GH Secretion. Neuroendocrinology, 1999, 69, 3-10.

Cassano PA *et al.* Obesity and body fat distribution in relation to the incidence of non-insulin-dependent diabetes mellitus. A prospective cohort study of men in the normative aging study. American Journal of Epidemiology, 1992, 136, 1474-1486.

Caterson ID. Obesity 1998—has anything changed? Mod Med Australia, 1998, 52-69.

Caterson ID. Obesity and its management. Australian Precriber, 1999, 22, 12-16.

Cefalu *et al.* The effect of chromium supplementation on carbohydrate and body fat distribution. Diabetes, 1997, 46(Suppl. 1), 55A

Chan JM *et al.* Obesity, fat distribution, and weight gain as riskfactors for clinical diabetes in men. Diabetes Care, 1994, 17, 961-969.

Chen H *et al.* Evidence that the diabetes gene encodes the leptin receptor: identification of a mutation in the leptin receptor gene in db/db mice. Cell 1996, 84, 491-495.

Chapman BJ, *et al.* The effects of a new b-adrenoceptor agonist BRL 26830A in refractory obesity. International Journal of Obesity, 1998 12, 119-123.

Ching PLYH, *et al.* Activity level and risk of overweight in male health professionals. Am Public Health, 1996, 86, 25-30.

Chisholm DJ, *et al.* Obesity: genes, glands or gluttony? Reprod Fertil Dev, 1998, 10(1), 49-53.

Chou P, *et al.* Associated risk factors of diabetes in Kin-Hu, Kinmen. Diabetes Res Clin Pract 1994, 26, 229-235.

Cinti S, *et al.* Immunoelectron microscopial identification of the uncoupling protein in brown adipose tissue mitochondria. Biology of the Cell, 1989, 67, 359-362.

Clancy SP *et al.* Effects of chromium picolinate supplementation on body composition, strength, and urinary chromium loss in football players. International Journal of Sport Nutrution, 1994, 4, 142-153.

Clinical Guidelines on the Identification, Evaluation, and Treatment of Overweight and Obesity in Adults. National Heart, Lung, and Blood Institute (NHLBI), Clinical Guidelines for Obesity, 1998.

Colditz GA. Economic costs of obesity. American Journal of Clinical Nutrition, 1992, 55, 503-507.

Connacher AA, *et al.* Metabolic effects of three weeks administration of b-adrenoceptor agonist BRL 26830A. International Journal of Obesity, 1992, 16, 685-694.

Connacher AA, *et al.* Weight loss in obese subjects on a restricted diet given BRL 26830A, a new atypical b adrenoceptor agonist. British Medical Journal, 1998, 296, 1217-1220.

Connoley IP, *et al.* Role of beta-adrenoceptors in mediating the thermogenic effects of sibutramine. British Journal of Pharmacology, 1996, 117, 170.

Connoley IP, *et al.* Thermogenic effects of sibutramine and its metabolites. British Journal of Pharmacology, 1999, 126, 1487-1495.

Connolly HM, *et al.* Valvular heart disease associated with fenfluramine-phentermine. New England Journal of Medicine, 1997, 337, 581-588

Davidson MH, *et al* Weight Control and Risk Factor Reduction in Obese Subjects Treated for 2 Years With Orlistat: A Randomized Controlled Trial. Journal of the American Medical Association, 1999, 281, 235-242.

Davidson MH *et al.* Weight control and risk factor reduction in obese subjects Journal of the American Medical Association, 1999, 20, 235-242.

Day C & Bailey CJ. Effect of the antiobesity agent sibutramine in obese-diabetic ob/ob mice. International Journal of Obesity and Related Metabolic Disorders 1998, 22, 619-623.

Deitel M & Petrov I. Incidence of symptomatic gallstones after bariatric operations. Surgery, Gynecology and Obstetrics, 1987, 164, 549-552.

Deitel M. Surgery for obesity—overview. European Journal of Gastroenterology and Hepatology, 1999, 11, 57-61.

Derôme-Tremblay M. History of dexfenfluramine. In: Obesity Management & Redux, Nicolaidis S (Ed). London: Academic Press, 1997.

Després JP *et al.* Regional distribution of body fat, plasma lipoproteins, and cardio-vascular disease. Arteriosclerosis, 1990, 10, 497-511.

Després JP. Abdominal obesity as important component of insulin-resistance syndrome. Nutrition, 1993, 9, 452-459.

Després JP. Dyslipidaemia and obesity. Baillieres Clin Endocrinol Metab, 1994, 8, 629-660.

DiPietro L Physical activity, body weight, and adiposity: an epidemiologic perspective. Exerc Sport Sciences Rev, 1995, 23, 275-303

Douglas NJ. The sleep apnoea/hypopnoea syndrome. European Journal of Clinical Investigations, 1995, 25, 285-290.

Dow RL. Beta-3 adrenergic agonists: potential therapeutics for obesity. Expert Opinion in Investigational Drugs, 1997, 6, 1811-1825.

Drent ML, *et al.* Orlistat (Ro 18-0647), a lipase inhibitor, in the treatment of human obesity: a multiple dose study. International Journal of Obesity and Related Metabolic Disorders, 1995, 4, 221-226.

Drent ML & van der Veen EA. First clinical studies with orlistat: a short review. Obesity Research, 1995, 3 (Suppl 4), 623S-625S.

Drent ML & van der Veen EA. Lipase inhibition: a novel concept in the treatment of obesity. International Journal of Obesity and Related Metabolic Disorders, 1993, 4, 241-244.

Drewnowski A, *et al.* Taste and eating disorders. American Journal of Clinical Nutrition, 1987, 46, 442-450.

Dunn AL, *et al.* Comparison of lifestyle and structured interventions to increase physical activity and cardiorespiratory fitness. Journal of the American Medical Association, 1999, 28, 327-334.

Dvorak R, *et al.* Drug therapy for obesity in the elderly. Drug Therapy, 1997, 11, 338-351.

Eighth International Congress on Obesity. Paris, France, 29 August-3 September 1998. Abstracts. International Journal of Obesity and Related Metabolic Disorders. 1998 Aug;22 (Suppl 3):S1-314.

Elchebly M *et al.* Increased insulin sensitivity and obesity resistance in mice lacking the protein tyrosine phosphatase-1B. Science, 1999, 283, 1544-1548.

Evans GW. The role of picolinic acid in metal metabolism. Life Chem Reports, 1982, 1, 57-67.

Evans GW. The effect of chromium picolinate on insulin controlled parameters in humans. Int J Biosoc Med Res, 1989, 11, 163-180.

Evans GW *et al.* Chromium picolinate decreases calcium excretion and increases dehydroepiandrosterone (DHEA) in postmenopausal womem. FASEB J, 1995, 9, 449A.

Everhart JE. Contributions of obesity and weight loss to gallstone disease. Annals of Internal Medicine, 1993, 119, 1029-1035.

Ezzell C. Leaping leptin. Scientific American, 1998. 279, 30.

Fantino M & Souguet A-M. Effects of metabolites 1 and 2 of sibutramine on the short-term control of food intake in the rat. International Journal of Obesity, 1995, 19, 145.

Felitti VJ. Childhood sexual abuse, depression, and family dysfunction in adult obese patients: a case control study. South Med J, 1993, 86, 732-736.

Felson DT & Chaisson CE. Understanding the relationship between body weight and osteoarthritis. Balliere's Clinical Rheumatology, 1997, 11, 671-681.

Ferrannini E *et al.* Hyperinsulinaemia: the key feature of a cardiovascular and metabolic syndrome. Diabetology, 1991, 34, 416-422.

Ferro-Luzzi A & Martino L. Obesity and physical activity. In:. The Origins and Consequences of Obesity, Chadwick D & Cardew G (Eds). Chichester: Wiley: 202-227, 1996.

Fink H, *et al.* Major biological actions of CCK-a critical evaluation of research findings. Exp Brain Res, 1998, 123, 77-83.

Finney LS *et al.* Dietary chromium and diabetes: Is there a relationship? Clin Diabetes, 1997, 15, 6.

Forrester T *et al.* Obesity in the Caibbean. Ciba Foundation Symposium, 1996, 201, 17-26.

Frühbeck G, *et al.* Leptin: physiology and pathophysiology. Clinical Physiology, 1998, 5, 399-419.

Gastric surgery for severe obesity. NIDDKD Publication No 96-4006, 1996.

Garfinkel L. Overweight and cancer. Annals of Internal Medicine, 1985, 103(6 Pt 2), 1034-1036.

Gill TP. Key issues in the prevention of obesity. British Medical Bulletin, 1997, 53, 359-388.

Glueck CJ, *et al.* Sucrose polyester: substitution for dietary fats in hypocaloric diets in the treatment of familial hypercholesterolaemia. American Journal of Clinical Nutrition, 1983, 37, 347-354.

Goran MI, *et al.* Longitudinal changes in fatness in white children: no effect of childhood energy expenditure. American Journal of Clinical Nutrition, 1998, 67, 309-316.

Goran MI. Variations in total energy expenditure in humans. Obesity Research, 1995, 3, 59-66.

Gorsky RD, *et al.* The 25-year health care costs of women who remain overweight after 40 years of age. American Journal of Preventive Medicine, 1996, 12, 388-394.

Gortmaker S, *et al.* Television viewing as a cause of increasing obesity among children in the United States. Arch Pediatr Adolesc Med, 1996, 150, 356-362.

Greenway FL. Clinical studies with phenylpropanolamine: a meta-analysis. American Journal of Clinical Nutrition, 1992, 55(Suppl 1), 203S-205S.

Griffiths M, *et al.* Metabolic rate and physical development in children at risk for obesity. Lancet, 1990, 336, 76-78.

Grippo JF & Burn P. Obesity genes: molecular genetic approaches to drug target identification. Il Farmaco, 1998, 53, 262-265.

Guerciolini R. Mode of action of orlistat. International Journal of Obesity, 1997, 21 (Suppl 3), S12-S23.

Gura T. Uncoupling Proteins Provide New Clue to Obesity's Causes. Science 1998, 280, 1369-1370.

Guy-Grand B. Pharmacological approaches to intervention. International Journal of Obesity, 1997, 21(Suppl 1), S22-S24.

Haffner SM. Risk factors for non-insulin-dependent diabetes mellitus. Journal of Hypertension (Suppl), 1995, 13, S73-S76.

Halaas JL, *et al.* Physiological response to long-term peripheral and central leptin infusion in leanand obese mice. Proc Natl Acad Sci USA, 1997, 94, 8878-8883.

Halaas JL, *et al.* Weight reducing effects of the plasma protein encoded by the obese gene. Science, 1995, 269, 543-546.

Han TS *et al.* Waist circumference relates to intra-abdominal fat mass better than waist-to-hip ratio in women. Proc Nutr Soc, 1995, 54(3), 152A.

Han TS *et al.* The influences of height and age on waist circumference as an index of adiposity in adults. International Journal of Obesity & Related Metabolic Diseases, 1997, 21, 83-89.

Han TS *et al.* Waist circumference reduction and cardiovascular benefits during weight loss in women. International Journal of Obesity & Related Metabolic Disorders, 1997, 21, 127-134.

Hanotin C *et al.* Comparison of sibutramine and dexfenfluramine in the treatment of obesity. Obesity Research, 1998, 6, 285-291.

Hanotin C *et al.* Efficacy and tolerability of sibutramine in obese patients: a dose-ranging study. International Journal of Obesity and Related Metabolic Disorders, 1998, 22, 32-38.

Hansen DL, *et al.* Thermogenic effects of sibutramine in humans. American Journal of Clinical Nutrition, 1998, 68, 1180-1186.

Hartmann D, *et al.* Influence of orlistat on the regulation of gallbladder contraction in man: a randomized double-blind placebo-controlled crossover study. Dig Dis Sci, 1996, 41, 2404-2408.

Hartmann D *et al.* Lack of interaction between orlistat and oral contraceptives. European Journal of Clinical Pharmacology, 1996, 50, 421-424.

Hartmann D, *et al.* Effect on dietary fat absorption of orlistat, administered at different times relative to meal intake. British Journal of Clinical Pharmacology, 1993, 36, 266-270.

Hartz AJ *et al.* The association of obesity with infertility and related menstrual abnormalities in women. International Journal of Obesity, 1979, 3, 57-73.

Healthy People 2000: National Health Promotion and Disease Preventive Objects. Washington DC: US Dept., of Health and Human Public Health Service: 1990: US Dept of Health and Human Services publication No. PHS 90-50212.

Herman CP, *et al.* Obesity, externality, and susceptibility to social influence: an integrated analysis. J Personal and Soc Psychol, 1983, 45, 926-934.

Herman J *et al.* Effects of chromium or copper supplementation on serum osteocalcin, parathyroid hormone, and alkaline phosphatase in adults over age 50. FASEB J, 1996, 10, 785A.

Heymsfield SB & Pietrobelli A. Morbid obesity: the price of progress. Endocr Pract, 1997, 3, 320-323.

Hill JO & Peters JC. Environmental Contributions to the Obesity Epidemic. Science, 1998, 280, 1371-1374.

Hill JO & Trowbridge FL. Childhood obesity: future directions and research priorities. Pediatrics, 1998, 1(Suppl. 3), 570-574.

Himms-Hagen J & Danforth E. The potential role of beta-3 adrenoceptor agonists in the treatment of obesity and diabetes. Current Opinion in Endocrionology & Diabetes, 1996, 3, 59-65.

Hoekenga MT, *et al.* A Comprehensive review of diethylpropion hydrochloride. In: Central Mechanisms of Anorectic Drugs. Garrattini S, Samanin R (Eds). New York: Raven, 1978.

Hollander PA, *et al.* Role of orlistat in the treatment of obese patients with type 2 diabetes. A 1-year randomized double-blind study. Diabetes Care, 1998, 8, 1288-1294.

Holley HS *et al.* Regional distribution of pulmonary ventilation and perfusion in obesity. Journal of Clinical Investigation, 1967, 46, 475-481.

Holst JJ. Glucagon-like peptide 1: a newly discovered gastrointestinal hormone. Gastroenterology, 1994, 107, 1848-1855.

Howard BV, *et al.* Studies of the etiology of obesity in Pima Indians. American Journal of Clinical Nutrition, 1991, 53, 1577S-1585S.

Huang Z, *et al.* Body weight, weight change, and risk for hypertension in women. Annals of Internal Medicine, 1998, 128, 81-88.

Huang Z, *et al.* Dual effects of weight and weight gain on breast cancer risk. Journal of the American Medical Association, 1997, 278, 1407-1411.

Hubert HB, *et al.* Obesity as an independent risk factor for cardiovascular disease: a 26-year follow-up of participants in the Framingham Heart Study. Circulation, 1983, 67, 968-977.

Huszonek J. Over the counter chromium picolinate (letter). American Journal of Psychiatry, 1993, 150, 1560-1561.

Ignjatovic V, *et al.* Clinical treatment of obesity using 'slimax' a traditional chinese medicine. In: Proceedings of the 8th International Congress on Obesity, Paris, France, 29 August—3 September 1998. Després J-P & Macdonald I (Eds): 22(Suppl 3);1998: S1-S314, Abstract P618, 1998.

Jack DB. Fighting obesity the Franco-British way. Lancet, 1996, 347, 1756.

Jackson RS *et al*. Obesity and impaired prohormone processing associated with mutations in the human prohormone convertase-1 gene. Nature Genetics, 1997, 16, 303-306.

James WP. The epidemiology of obesity. In: The Origins and Consequences of Obesity. Chadwick D, Cardew G (Eds). Chichester: Wiley, 1-16, 1996.

James WP, *et al*. A one-year trial to assess the value of orlistat in the management of obesity. International Journal of Obesity and Related Metabolic Disorders, 1997, 21(Suppl 3), S24-30.

James WP et al.: Effect of sibutramine on weight maintenance after weight loss: a randomised trial. STORM Study Group. Sibutramine Trial of Obesity Reduction and Maintenance. Lancet 356:21;19-25.

Jebb SA. Aetiology of obesity. British Medical Bulletin, 1997, 53(No.2), 264-285.

Jebb SA, *et al*. Obesity and social class in women: effects of smoking, drinking and physical activity. Proc Nutr Soc, 1997, 56(1A), 159A.

Jones PJH, Kitts DD. How the body uses fat. Nutr Quart, 1994, 18, 93-101.

Jung RT. Obesity as a disease. British Medical Bulletin, 1997, 53, 307-321.

Kadowaki H *et al*. A mutation on the beta-3-adrenergic receptor gene is associated with obesity and hyperinsulinaemia in Japanese subjects. Biochemical and Biophysical Research Communications, 1995, 215, 555-560.

Karlsson C, *et al*. Effects of growth hormone treatment on the leptin system and on energy expenditure in abdominally obese men. European Journal of Endocrinology, 1998, 138, 408-414.

Karp WB. Childhood and adolescent obesity: a national epidemic.
Journal of the Californian Dental Association, 1998, 26, 771-773.

Keightly PD. Chewing the fat. Nature Genetics, 1995, 10, 125-126.

Kiberstis PA & Marx J. Regulation of Body Weight. Science, 1998, 280, 1363.

King DJ & Devaney N. Clinical pharmacology of sibutramine hydrochloride (BTS 54524), a new antidepressant, in healthy volunteers. British Journal of Clinical Pharmacology, 1998, 26, 607-611.

Kirkland JL & Hollenberg CH. Inhibitors of preadipocyte replication: opportunities for the treatment of obesity. Prog Mol Sub Biol, 1998, 20, 177-195.

Kissebah AH *et al*. Health risks of obesity. Medical Clinics of North Americs, 1989, 73, 111-138.

Klaus S, *et al*. The uncoupling protein UCP: a membraneous mitochondrial ion carrier exclusively expressed in brown adipose tissue. International Journal of Biochemistry, 1991, 23, 791-801.

Klebig ML *et al*. Ectopic expression of the agouti gene in transgenic mice causes obesity, features type II diabetes, yellow fur. Proceedings of the National Academy of Sciences of the USA, 1995, 92, 4728-4732.

Klesges RC, *et al*. A longitudinal analysis of the impact of dietary intake and physical activity on weight change in adults. American Journal of Clinical Nutrition, 1992, 55, 818-822.

Kleyn PW, *et al*. Identification and characterisation of the mouse obesity gene tubby: a member of a novel gene family. Cell, 1996, 85, 281-290.

Knopp RH *et al*. A double-blind randomised, controlled trial of the effects of two eggs per day in moderately hypercholesterolemic and combined hyperlipidemic subjects taught the NCEP step I diet. Journal of the American College of Nutrition, 1997, 16, 551-561.

Kopelman PG. Hormones and obesity. Baillieres Clin Endocrinol Metab, 1994, 8, 549-575

Kortt MA, *et al*. A review of cost-of-illness studies on obesity. Clin Therap, 1998, 20, 772-779.

Kuczmarski RJ, *et al*. Increasing prevalence of overweight among US adults: the National Health and Nutrition Examination Surveys, 1960-1991. Journal of the American Medical Association, 1994, 272, 205-211.

Kuller LH. The etiology of breast cancer-from epidemiology to prevention. Public Health Review, 1995, 23, 157-213.

Kumanyika S. Ethnicity and obesity development in children. Ann N Y Acad Sci, 1993, 699, 81

Kurscheid T & Lauterbach K. The cost implications of obesity for health care and society. International Journal of Obesity and Related Metabolic Disorders, 1998, 22(Suppl 1), S3-S5.

Laloi M, *et al*. A plant cold-induced uncoupling protein. Nature, 1997, 389,135-136.

Landsberg L. Pathophysiology of obesity-related hypertension: role of insulin and the sympathetic nervous system. J Cardiovasc Pharmacol, 1994, 23(Suppl 1), S1-S8.

Lapidus L *et al*. Distribution of adipose tissue and risk of cardiovascular disease and death: a twelve year follow up of participants in the population study of women in Gothenburg, Sweden. British Medical Journal, 1984, 289, 1257-1261.

Larson DE, *et al.*Energy metabolism in weight-stable postobese individuals. American Journal of Clinical Nutrition, 1995, 62, 735-739.

Larsson B *et al.* Abdominal adipose tissue distribution, obesity, and risk of cardiovascular disease and death: 13 year follow-up of participants in the study of men born in 1913. Br Med J Clin Res, 1984, 288, 1401-1404.

Le Riche WH & Csima A. A long-acting appetite suppressant drug studied for 24 weeks in both continuous and sequential administration. Canadian Medical Association Journal, 1967, 97, 1016-1020.

Lean MEJ, et al. Predicting body composition by densitometry from simple anthropometric measurements. American Journal of Clinical Nutrition, 1996, 63, 4-14.

Lean MEJ. Sibutramine—a review of clinical efficacy. International Journal of Obesity and Related Metabolic Disorders, 1997, 21(Suppl 1), S30-36.

Lean MEJ, *et al.* Waist circumference as a measure for indicating need for weight management. British Medical Journal, 1995, 311, 158-161.

Lee IM, *et al.* Body weight and mortality: a 27-year follow-up of middle-aged men. Journal of the American Medical Association, 1993, 270, 2823-2828.

Lee NA. Beneficial effect of chromium supplementation on serum triglyceride levels in NIDDM. Diabetes Care, 1994, 17, 1449-1452.

Lefavi RG. Sizing up a few supplements. Physical Sports Medicine, 1992, 20,191-191.

Levy E, *et al.* The economic cost of obesity: The French situation. International Journal of Obesity and Related Metabolic Disorders, 1995, 19, 788-792.

Lew EA & Garfinkel L. Variations in mortality by weight among 750,000 men and women. Journal of Chronic Disorders, 1979, 32, 563-576.

Liu Y-L *et al.* Contribution of B3-adrenoceptor activation to ephedrine-induced thermogenesis in humans. International Journal of Obesity, 1995, 19, 678-685.

Louis P, *et al.* The human obesity gene map: the 1998 update. Obesity Research, 1999, 111-129

Lowell BB & Flier JS. Brown adipose tissue, beta-3 adrenergic receptors and obesity. Annual Review Medicine, 1997, 48, 307-316.

Lowell B, *et al.* Development of obesity in transgenic mice after genetic ablation of brown adipose tissue. Nature, 1993, 366, 740-742.

Lukaski HC *et al.* Chromium supplementation and resistance training: effects on body composition, strength, and trace element status of men. American Journal of Clinical Nutrition, 1996, 63, 954-965.

Lundgren H *et al.* Adiposity and adipose tissue distribution in relation to incidence of diabetes in women: results from a prospective population study in Gothenburg, Sweden. International Journal of Obesity, 1989, 13, 413-423.

Maclure KM *et al.* Weight, diet, and the risk of symptomatic gallstones in middle-aged women. New England Journal of Medicine, 1989, 321, 563-569.

Malchow-Møller A, *et al.* Ephedrine as an anorectic: the story of the 'Elsinore pill'. International Journal of Obesity, 1981, 5, 183-188.

Marcus MD, Wing RR, Ewing L *et al.* A double-blind, placebo-controlled trial of flu-oxetine plus behaviour modification in the treatment of obese binge-eaters and non-binge-eaters. American Journal of Psychiatry, 1990, 147, 876-881.

Marks BL, *et al.* Fat-free mass is maintained in women following a moderate diet and exercise program. Med Sci Sports Exerc, 1995, 27, 1243-1251.

Marlatt GA & Gordon J. Relapse prevention: maintenance strategies in addictive behaviour change. New York: Guildford, 1985.

McCann B, *et al.* Changes in plasma lipids and dietary intake accompanying shifts in perceived workload and stress. Psychosomatic Medicine, 1990, 52, 97-108.

McCarty MF. Anabolic effects of insulin on bone suggest a role for chromium picoli-nate in preservation of bone density. Med Hypotheses, 1995, Set 45, 241-246.

McKeigue PM *et al.* Relationship of glucose intolerance and hyperinsulinaemia to body fat patterns in south Asians and Europeans. Diabetologia, 1992, 35, 785-791.

McGinnis JM & Foege WH. Actual causes of death in the United States. Journal of the American Medical Association, 1993, 270, 2207-2212.

McNeely W &Benfield P. Orlistat. Drugs, 1998, 56(2), 241-250.

McNeely W & Goa KL. Sibutramine: A Review of its Contribution to the Management of Obesity. Drugs, 1999, 56, 1093-1124.

Mejean A, *et al.* Carazolol: a potent selective β_3-adrenergic receptor agonist. European Journal of Pharmacolology, 1995, 291, 359-366.

Melia AT, *et al.* Retrospective population-based analysis of the dose-response (fecal fat excretion) relationship of orlistat in normal and obese volunteers. Clin Pharmacol Ther, 1994, 56, 82-85.

Melia AT *et al.* The influence of reduced dietary fat absorption induced by orlistat on the pharmacokinetics of digoxin in healthy volunteers. Journal of Clinical Pharmacology, 1995, 35, 840-843.

Melia AT *et al.* Lack of effect of orlistat on the bioavailability of a single dose of nifedipin extended-release tablets (Procardia XL) in healthy volunteers. Journal of Clinical Pharmacology, 1996, 36, 352-355.

Melia AT *et al.* The effect of orlistat, an inhibitor of dietary fat absorption, on the absorption of vitamins A and E in healthy volunteers. Journal of Clinical Pharmacology, 1996, 36, 647-653.

Melia AT *et al.*The effect of orlistat on the pharmacokinetics of phenytoin in healthy volunteers. Journal of Clinical Pharmacology, 1996, 36, 654-658.

Melia AT, *et al.* Review of limited systemic absorption of orlistat, a lipase inhibitor, in healthy human volunteers. Journal of Clinical Pharmacology, 1995, 35, 1103-1108.

Metropolitan Life Foundation. Metropolitan height and weight tables. Statistical Bulletin, 1983, 64, 2-9.

Mincheva V, *et al.* Bee products as a potential treatment of obesity. In: Proceedings of the 8th International Congress on Obesity, Paris, France, 29 August—3 September 1998. Després J-P & Macdonald I (Eds): 22(Suppl 3),S1-S314, Abstract P617, 1998.

Montague CT, *et al.* Congenital leptin deficiency is associated with severe early-onset obesity in humans. Nature, 1997, 387, 903-908.

Mrad AJ, *et al.* Skeletal muscle composition in dietary obesity-susceptible and dietary obesity-resistant rats. American Journal of Physiology, 1992, 262, R684-R688.

Musaiger A. Trends in diet-related chronic diseases in United Arab Emirates. In: Musaiger AO, Miladi SS (Eds). Diet-related non-communicable diseases in the Arab countries of the Gulf. Cairo, Food and Agriculture Organization of the United Nations, 1996, 99-117.

Mussell M, *et al.* Onset of binge eating, dieting, obesity and mood disorders among subjects seeking treatment for binge eating disorder. International Journal of Eating Disorders, 1995, 17, 395-401.

Must A, Jacques PF, Dallal GE *et al.* Long-term morbidity and mortality of overweight adolescents: a follow up of the Harvard Growth Study of 1922-1935. New England Journal of Medicine, 1992, 327, 1350.

Naggert JK, *et al.* Hyperproinsulinaemia in obese fat/fat mice associated with a carboxypeptidase E mutation which reduces enzyme activity. Nature Genetics, 1995, 10, 135-142.

Nagle DL, McGrail SH, Vitale J, *et al.* The *mahogany* protein is a receptor involved in suppression of obesity. Nature, 1999, 11, 148-152.

Nairnark X & Cherniak RM. Compliance of the respiratory system and its components in health and obesity. Journal of Applied Physiology, 1960, 15, 377-382.

Nakajima T, *et al..* Noninvasive study of left ventricular performance in obese patients: influence of duration on obesity. Circulation, 1985, 71, 481-486.

National Academy of Sciences. Diet and health. Washington DC: National Academy of Science Press, 1991.

National Heart, Lung and Blood Institute. Clinical guidelines on the identification, evaluation, and treatment of overweight and obesity in adults, 1998.

National Task Force on the Prevention of Obesity. Long-term pharmacotherapy in the management of obesity. Journal of the American Medical Association, 1996, 276, 907-1915.

Nelson KM, *et al*. Prediction of energy expenditure from fat-free mass and fat mass. American Journal of Clinical Nutrition, 1992, 56, 848-856.

Nelson KM, *et al*. Effect of weight reduction on resting energy expenditure, substrate utilization, and the thermic effect of food in moderately obese women. American Journal of Clinical Nutrition, 1992, 55, 924-933.

Newman BY. Guidelines on obesity. J Am Optom Assoc, 1998, 69, 688.

Niijima A, *et al*. Role of ventrohypothalamus on sympathetic efferent of brown adipose tissue. American Journal of Physiology 1984, 247, R650-R654.

Nishikawa T, *et al*. Effect of mazindol on body weight and insulin sensitivityin severely obese patients after a very low calorie diet therapy. Endocrinology Journal, 1996, 43, 671-677.

Noben-Trauth K *et al*. A candidate gene for the mouse mutation tubby. Nature, 1996, 380, 534-538.

Ohlson LO *et al*. The influence of body fat distribution on the incidence of diabetes mellitus. 13.5 years of follow up of the participants in the study of men born in 1913. 1985, 34, 1055-1058.

Onishi T. Clinical evaluation of mazindol, an anorexiant on obesity. International Journal of Obesity, 1990, 14(Suppl 2), 34.

O'Shea D, *et al*. Neuropeptide Y induced feeding in the rat is mediated by a novel receptor. Endocrinology, 1997, 138, 196-202.

Paez X & Myers RD. Insatiable feeding evoked in rats by recurrent perfusion of neuropeptide Y in the hypothalamus. Peptides, 1991, 12, 609-616.

Parisi AF. Diet-drug debacle. Annals of Internal Medicine, 1998, 129, 903-905.

Pasquali R & Casimirri F. The impact of obesity on hyperandrogenism and polycystic ovary syndrome in premenopausal women. Clinical Endocrinology (Oxf), 1993, 39, 1-16.

Peeke PM & Chrousos GP. Hypercortisolism and obesity. Ann N Y Acad Sci., 1995, 771, 665-676

Pellymounter M, *et al.* Effects of the obese gene product on body weight regulation in ob/ob mice. Science, 1995, 269, 540-542.

Perri MG & Fuller PR. Success and failure in the treatment of obesity: where do we go from here? Med Exerc Nutr Health. 1995, 4, 255-272.

Pette D & Spamer C. Metabolic properties of muscle fibers. Fed Proc 1986, 4, 2910-2914.

Pishdad GR. Overweight and obesity in adults aged 20-74 in southern Iran. International Journal of Obesity and Related Metabolic Disorders, 1996, 20, 963-965.

Pi-Sunyer FX. Medical hazards of obesity. Annals of Internal Medicine, 1993, 119, 655-660.

Plotsky PM, *et al.* Hypothalamic-pituitary-adrenal axis function in the Zucker obese rat. Endocrinology, 1992, 130, 1931-1941.

Position of the American Dietetic Association: medical nutrition therapy and pharmacotherapy. Journal of the American Dietetic Associaton, 1999, 99, 227-30.

Prevention of obesity: Berzelius Symposium 42 (1998). Satellite Symposium of the 8th International Congress of Obesity. Swedish Society of Medicine, Stockholm. 26-28 August 1998. Appetite, Dec;31(3):407-436.

Prouix LG. Diet drugs at a glance. Washington Post Health Supplement. September 16, 1997, 13 (col 3).

Ravussin E & Swinburn BA. Pathophysiology of obesity. Lancet, 1992, 340, 404-408.

Ravussin E, *et al.* Reduced rate of energy expenditure as a risk factor for body weight gain. New England Journal of Medicine, 1988, 318, 467-472.

Ravussin E & Swinburn BA. Metabolic predictors of obesity. Cross-sectional versus longitudinal data. International Journal of Obesity, 1993, 17, S28-S31.

Ravussin E. Metabolic differences and the development of obesity. Metabolism, 1995, 9(Suppl. 3), 12-14.

Raymond NR & D'Eramo-Melkus G. Non-insulin-dependent diabetes and obesity in the black and Hispanic population: culturally sensitive management. Diabetes Educ, 1993, 19, 313-317.

Report of a WHO Consultation on Obesity: Obesity—Preventing and Managing the Global Epidemic. World Health Organization, June 3-5, 1997.

Ricquier D, *et al.* (Expression of uncoupling protein mRNA in thermogenic or weakly thermogenic brown adipose tissue. Evidence for a rapid beta-adrenoreceptor-mediated and transcriptionally regulated step during activation of thermogenesis. J Biol Chem, 1986, 261, 13905-13910.

Rippe JM & Hess S. The role of physical activity in the prevention and managemnet of obesity. Journal of the American Dietetic Association, 1998, 98(Suppl 2), S31-S38.

Rissanen AM, et al. Determinants of weight gain and overweight in adult Finns. European Journal of Clinical Nutrition, 1991, 45, 419-430.

Roberts SB, et al. Energy expenditure and intake in infants born to lean and over-weight mothers. New England Journal of Medicine, 1988, 318, 461-466.

Rohner-Jeanrenaud F & Jeanrenaud B. Acute intravenous corticotropin-releasing factor administration: effects on insulin secretion in lean and genetically obese fa/fa rats. Endocrinology, 1992, 130, 1903-1908.

Rolls BJ & Snide DJ. The influence of dietary fat on food intake and body weight. Nutr Rev, 1992, 50, 283-290.

Rolls BJ. Carbohydrate, fats and satiety. American Journal of Clinical Nutrition, 1995, 61, 960-967.

Rössner S et al: Weight loss, weight maintenance, and improved cardiovascular risk factors after 2 years treatment with orlistat for obesity. European Orlistat Obesity Study Group. Obesity Research 2000; 8:49-61

Ryan DH, et al. Sibutramine: a novel new agent for obesity treatment. Obesity Research, 1995, 3(Suppl 4), 553S-559S.

Safer DJ. Diet, behaviour modification, and exercise: a review of obesity treatments from a long-term perspective. Southern Medical Journal, 1991, 84, 1470-1474.

Sargent PA, et al. 5-HT$_{2C}$ receptor activation decreases appetite and body weight in obese subjects. Psychopharmacology, 1997, 133, 309-312.

Saris WHM. Fit, fat and fat free: the metabolic aspects of weight control. International Journal of Obesity, 1998, 22(Suppl 2), S15-S21.

Saw SM & Rajan U. The epidemiology of obesity: a review. Ann Acad Med Singapore, 1997, 26, 489-493.

Sayler ME, et al. Evaluating success of weight loss programs, with an application to fluoxetine weight reduction clinical trial data. International Journal of Obesity and Related Metabolic Disorders, 1994, 18, 742-751.

Schachter S. Some extraordinary facts about obese humans and rats. American Psychologist, 1971, 26, 129-144.

Schwartz MR, et al. Insulin in the brain : a hormonal regulator of energy balance. Endocrinology Reviews, 1992, 13, 387-414.

Schonfeld-Warden N, Warden CH. Pediatric obesity: An overview of etiology and treatment. Pediatric Endocrinology, 1997, 44, 339-361.

Scottish Intercollegiate Guidelines Network. The management of obese patients in Scotland: a new approach in primary health care with a national prevention and management strategy. Edinburgh, 1996.

Seagle HM, et al. Effects of sibutramine on resting metabolic rate and weight loss in overweight women. Obesity Research, 1998, 6, 115-121

Seeley RJ et al. Melanocortin receptors in leptin effects. Nature, 1997, 390, 349.

Segal L, et al. The cost of obesity. The Australian perspective. PharmacoEconomics, 1994, 5(Suppl 1), 45-52.

Seidell JC. The impact of obesity on health status: some implications for health care costs. International Journal of Obesity and Related Metabolic Disorders, 1995, 19, S13-S16.

Seidell JC, et al. Fasting respiratory exchange ratio and resting metabolic rate as predictors of weight gain: the Baltimore Longitudinal Study on Aging. International Journal of Obesity, 1992, 16, 667-674.

Seidell JC. Time trends in obesity: an epidemiological perspective. Horm Metab Res, 1997, 155-158

Seidell JC. Societal and personal costs of obesity. Exp Clin Endocrinol Diabetes, 1998, 106, 7-9.

Seidell JC, et al. Body fat distribution in relation to physical activity and smoking habits in 38-year old European men. American Journal of Epidemioliology, 1991, 133, 257-265.

Shahi B et al. Sleep-related disorders in the obese. Obesity Surgery, 1992, 2, 157-168.

Sipols AJ, et al. Effect of intracerebroventricular insulin infusion on diabetic hyperphagia and hypothalamic neuropeptide gene expression. Diabetes, 1994, 44, 147-151.

Sjöström L, et al. Randomised placebo-controlled trial of orlistat for weight loss and prevention of weight regain in obese patients. European Multicentre Orlistat Study Group. Lancet, 1998, 352, 167-172.

Skarfors ET, et al. Risk factors for developing non-insulin dependent diabetes: a 10-year follow-up of men in Uppsala. British Medical Journal, 1991, 303, 755-760

Smith GP, Gibbs FP. Satiating effects of cholecystokinin. In: Annals of the New York Academy of Sciences: Cholecystokinin. Reeve JRJ, Eysselein V, Solomon TE, Go VLW (Eds). New York: New York Academy of Sciences, 1994, 236-241.

Sours HE, et al. Sudden death associated with very low calorie weight reduction regimens. American Journal of Clinical Nutrition, 1981, 34, 453-461.

Spiegel T, et al. Responses of lean and obese subjects to preloads, deprivation and palatibility. Appetite, 1989, 13, 45-69.

Spitzer L & Rodin J. Human eating behaviour: a critical review of studies in normal weight and overweight individuals. Appetite, 1981, 2, 293-329.

Statement of the American College of Cardiology on recommendations for patients who have used anorectic drugs. 18 October 1997. http://www.acc.org/pubs/news/statement.html

Stearns DM, et al. Chromium (III) picolinate produces chromosome damage in Chinese hamster ovary cells. FASEB J, 1995, 9, 1643-1648.

Steinbach G, et al. Effect of caloric restriction on colonic proliferation in obese persons: implications for colon cancer prevention. Cancer Research, 1994, 54, 1194-1197.

Steyn K et al. Risk factors for coronary heart disease in the Black population of the Cape Peninsula. South African Medical Journal, 1991, 79, 480-485.

Stock MJ. Sibutramine: a review of the pharmacology of a novel antiobesity agent. International Journal of Obesity and Related Metabolic Disorders, 1997, 21(Suppl 1) S25-59.

Strollo PJ Jr & Rogers RM. Current concepts: obstructive sleep apnoea. New England Journal of Medicine, 1996, 334, 99-104.

Sugerman HJ et al. Gastric bypass for treating severe obesity. American Journal of Clinical Nutrition, 1992, 55 (Suppl 2), S605-S665.

Svensson J, et al..: Two-month treatment of obese subjects with the oral growth hormone (GH) secretagogue MK-677 increases GH secretion, fat-free mass, and energy expenditure. Journal of Clinical Endocrinology and Metabolism, 1998, 83, 362-369.

Swinburn B, et al. Health care costs of obesity in New Zealand. International Journal of Obesity and Related Metabolic Disorders, 1997, 21, 891-896.

Swinburn BA et al. Body composition differences between Polynesians and Caucasians assessed by bioelectrical impedance. International Journal of Obesity & Related Metabolic Diseases, 1996, 20, 889-894.

Tartaglia L et al. Identification and expression cloning of a leptin receptor, OB-R. Cell, 1995, 83, 1263-1271.

Tataranni PA, Young JB, Bogardus C, et al. A low sympathoadrenal activity is associated with body weight gain and development of central adiposity in Pima Indian men. Obesity Research, 1997, 5, 341-347.

Tataranni PA. From physiology to neuroendocrinology: a reappraisal of risk factors of body weight gain in humans, 1998, 23, 108-115.

Tataranni PA & Ravussin E. Variability in metabolic rate: biological sites of regulation. International Journal of Obesity, 1995, 19, S101-S106.

Taubes G. As Obesity Rates Rise, Experts Struggle to Explain Why. Science, 1998 280, 1367-1368.

Taubes G. Weight Increases Worldwide?.Science, 1998, 280, 1368.

The Causes and Health Consequences of Obesity in Children and Adolescents: Hill JO & Trowbridge FL (Eds). Pediatrics, 101(Suppl 3), 497-574.

The management of obese patients in Scotland: integrating a new approach in primary health care with a national prevention and management strategy (1996). Edinburgh: Scottish Intercollegiate Guidelines Network.

The Obesity Epidemic: A Mandate for a Multidisciplinary Approach. Rippe JM (Ed). Journal of the American Dietetic Association. 1998, 98(Suppl. 2), S5-S64.

The Obesity Epidemic: A Mandate for a Multidisciplinary Approach (1998) Proceedings of a roundtable. Boston, Massachusetts, USA. October 27, 1997. Journal of the American Dietetic Association, October 1998, 10 Suppl 2, S1-61.

Thiele TE, *et al.* Central infusion of melanocortin agonist MTII in rats: assessment of c-Fos expression and taste aversion. American Journal of Physiology, 1998, 274(1 Pt 2), R248-54.

Thorburn AW & Proietto J. Neuropeptides, the hypothalamus and obesity: insights into the central control of body weight. Pathology, 1998, 30, 229-236.

Thurlby PL & Ellis RDM. Differences between the effects of noradrenaline and the b-adrenoceptor agonist BRL 28410 in brown adipose tissue and hind limb of the anaes-thetised rat. Canadian Journal of Physiology and Pharmacology, 1985, 64, 1111-1114.

Tremblay A, *et al.* Effect of intensity of physical activity on body fatness and fat distri-bution. American Journal of Clinical Nutrition, 1990, 51, 153-157.

Troiano RP, *et al.* Overweight prevalence and trends for children and adolescents: The National Health and Nutrition Examination Surveys, 1963-1991. Arch Pediatr Adolesc Med, 1995, 149, 1085.

Troisi RJ, *et al.* Cigarette smoking, dietary intake and physical activity : effects on body fat distribution—the Normative Aging Study. American Journal of Clinical Nutrition, 1991, 53, 1104-1111.

Tremblay A, *et al.* Effect of intensity of physical activity on body fatness and fat distri-bution. American Journal of Clinical Nutrition, 1990, 51, 153-157.

Tucker LA & Kano M. Dietary fat and body fat: a multivariate study of 205 adult females. American Journal of Clinical Nutrition, 1992, 56, 616-622.

Turton MD, *et al.* A role for glucagon-like peptide 1 in the central regulation of feed-ing. Nature, 1996, 379, 69-72.

Van Gaal,LF *et al.* Sibutramine and fat distribution: is there a role for pharmacotherapy in abdominal/visceral fat reduction? International Journal of Obesity and Related Metabolic Disorders, 1998, 22(Suppl 1), S38-40

Van Gaal LF, *et al.* Efficacy and tolerability of orlistat in the treatment of obesity: a 6-month dose-ranging study. Orlistat Dose-Ranging Study Group. European Journal of Clinical Pharmacology, 1998, 54, 125-132.

Van Heek M, *et al.* Diet-induced obese mice develop peripheral, but not central, resistance, to leptin. Journal of Clinical Investigations, 1997, 99, 385-390.

Van Itallie TB. Health implications of overweight and obesity in the United States. Annals of Internal Medicine, 1985, 103(6 Pt 2), 983-988.

Venne-Verboeket WV, *et al.* Effect of the pattern of food intake on human energy metabolism. British Journal of Nutrition, 1993, 70, 103-115.

Vgontzas AN *et al.* Sleep apnoea and sleep disruption in obese patients. Archives of Internal Medicine, 154, 1994, 1705-1711.

Villa P, *et al..* Impact of long-term naltrexone treatment on growth hormone and insulin secretion in hyperandrogenic and normal obese patients. Metabolism, 1997, 46, 538-543.

Wadden TA, *et al.* Sertraline and relapse prevention training following treatment by very low calorie diet: a controlled clinical trial. Obesity Research, 1995, 3, 549-558.

Wade AJ,*et al.* Muscle fibre type and aetiology of obesity. Lancet, 1990, 335, 805-808.

Walker ARP. Epidemiology and health inmplications in Southern Africa. In: Fourie J, Steyn S (Eds). Chronic diseases of lifestyle in South Africa: review of research and identification of essential health research priority. Parrow, Cape Town, Medical Research Council, 1995, 73-85.

Walsh BT & Devlin MJ. Eating Disorders: Progress and Problems. Science, 1998, 280, 1387-1390.

Wasser WG, *et al.* Chronic renal failure after ingestion of over the counter chromium picolinate. Annals of Internal Medicine, 1997, 126, 410.

Walston J, *et al.* A missense mutation in the B3-adrenergic receptor gene in Pima Indians and other populations with obesity and diabetes mellitus. New England Journal of Medicine, 1995, 333, 343-347.

Weintraub M, *et al.* Long-term weight control: the National Heart, Lung and Blood Institute funded multimodal intervention study. Clinical Pharmacol Ther, 1992, 51(Suppl 5), 581-646.

Weber C et *al*. Effect of the lipase inhibitor orlistat on the pharmacokinetics of four different antihypertensive drugs in healthy volunteers. European Journal of Clinical Pharmacology, 1996, 51, 87-90.

Weinsier RL, *et al*. Metabolic predictors of obesity: contributions of resting energy expenditure, thermic effect of food, and fuel utilization to four-year weight gain of post-obese and never-obese women. Journal of Clinical Investigation, 1995, 95, 980-985.

Weinsier RL, *et al*. The etiology of obesity: relative contribution of metabolic factors, diet, and physical activity. American Journal of Medicine, 1998, 105, 145-150.

Weintraub M, *et al*. Sibutramine in weight control: a dose-ranging, efficacy study. Clin Pharmacol Ther, 1991, 50, 330-337.

WHO MONICA Project. Geographical variation in the major risk factors of coronary heart disease in men and women aged 35-64 years. World Health Statistics Quarterly, 1988, 41, 115-140

WHO MONICA Project. Risk Factors. International Journal of Epidemiology, 1989, 18(Suppl. 1), S46-S55.

Wickelgren I. Do 'Apples' Fare Worse Than 'Pears'?. Science, 1998 280.

Wickelgren I. Obesity: How Big a Problem?.Science, 1998, 280, 1364-1367

Wigand R, *et al*. New human adenovirus (candidate adenovirus 36), a novel member of subgroup D. Archives of Virology, 1980, 64, 225-233.

Wilks R, *et al*. Obesity in peoples of the African diaspora. In: The Origins and Consequences of Obesity. Chadwick D & Cardew G (Eds). Chichester: Wiley: 37-53, 1996.

Willett WC. Dietary fat: an unconvincing relation. American Journal of Clinical Nutrition, 68, 1998, 1149-1150.

Williamson DF, *et al*. Recreational physical activity and 10-year weight change in a US national cohort. International Journal of Obesity, 1993, 17, 279-286.

Wolf AM. What is the economic case for treating obesity? Obesity Research, 1998, 6, 2S-7S

Wolf AM & Colditz GA. Social and economic effects of body weight in the United States. American Journal of Clinical Nutrition, 1996, 63, 466S-469S

Wolf AM & Colditz GA. Current estimates of the economic cost of obesity in the United States. Obesity Research, 1998, 6, 97-106.

Wolf AM. What is the economic cost for treating obesity? Obesity Research, 1998, 6, 2S-7S.

Wood P, *et al.* Changes in plasma lipids and lipoproteins in overweight men during weight loss through dieting as compared with exercise. New England Journal of Medicine, 1988, 319, 1173-1179.

Woods SC, *et al.* Signals That Regulate Food Intake and Energy Homeostasis. Science, 1998, 280, 1378-1383.

Yang H, *et al.* Risk factors for gallstone formation during rapid loss of weight. Dig Dis Sci, 1992, 37, 912-918.

Young *et al.* Prospective study of relative weight and risk of breast cancer: the Breast Cancer Detection Demonstration Project follow-up study, 1979 to 1987-1989. American Journal of Epidemiology, 1996, 143, 985-995.

Zemel MB. Insulin resistance, obesity and hypertension: an overview. Journal of Nutrition, 1995, 125(Suppl 6), 1715S-1717S.

Zhang *et al.* Positional cloning of the mouse obese gene and its human homologue. Nature 1994, 372, 425-432.

Zhi J, *et al.* Retrospective population-based analysis of the dose-response (fecal fat excretion) relationship of orlistat in normal and obese volunteers. Clin Pharmacol Ther, 1994, 56, 82-85.

Zhi J *et al.* The influence of orlistat on the pharmacokinetics and pharmacodynamics of glyburide in healthy volunteers. Journal of Clinical Pharmacology, 1995, 35, 521-525.

Zhi J *et al.* The effect of orlistat, an inhibitor of dietary fat absorption, on the pharmacokinetics of beta-carotene in healthy volunteers. Journal of Clinical Pharmacology, 1996, 36, 152-159.

Zhi J, *et al.* Review of limited systemic absorption Xenical, a lipase inhibitor, in healthy human volunteers. Journal of Clinical Pharmacology, 1995, 35, 1103-1108.

Zurlo F, *et al.* Low ratio of fat to carbohydrate oxidation as predictor of weight gain: study of 24-hRQ. American Journal of Physiology, 1990, 259, E650-E657.

ABOUT THE AUTHOR

Tim Atkinson is an established scientist and biomedical writer who has written numerous lectures, books, news features and scientific articles over a 10-year period. He also practices as a healthcare analyst who has published over a dozen management reports for the medical and pharmaceutical profession. He has an interest in the psychology of health, lifestyle disorders, stress and its effects on the immune system, and the effects of physical activity on the body, as well as being a personal fitness and bodybuilding trainer.

0-595-34916-1